PERFORMANCE INCENTIVES FOR GLOBAL HEALTH

PERFORMANCE INCENTIVES FOR GLOBAL HEALTH

Potential and Pitfalls

Rena Eichler, Ruth Levine, and the
Performance-Based Incentives Working Group

CENTER FOR GLOBAL DEVELOPMENT
Washington, D.C.

Performance Incentives for Global Health: Potential and Pitfalls may be ordered from:
BROOKINGS INSTITUTION PRESS
c/o HFS, P.O. Box 50370, Baltimore, MD 21211-4370
Tel.: 800/537-5487; 410/516-6956; Fax: 410/516-6998; Internet: www.brookings.edu

Library of Congress Cataloging-in-Publication data
Eichler, Rena.
  Performance incentives for global health : potential and pitfalls / Rena Eichler, Ruth
Levine and the Performance-Based Incentives Working Group.
       p. ;   cm.
  Includes bibliographical references.
  Summary: "Describes the rationale for introducing incentives tied to achievement of spe-
cific health-related targets, and provides guidance about designing, implementing, and eval-
uating programs that provide incentives to health care providers and patients. Presents case
studies that focus on recent uses of incentives addressing a range of health conditions in
diverse countries"—Provided by publisher.
  ISBN 978-1-933286-29-7 (pbk. : alk. paper)
  1. Medical economics. 2. World health. 3. Health promotion. I. Levine, Ruth, 1959– II.
Center for Global Development. Performance-Based Incentives Working Group. III. Title.
  [DNLM: 1. Delivery of Health Care—economics. 2. Program Evaluation—economics. 3.
Reimbursement, Incentive—economics. 4. World Health. W 84.1 P4376 2009]
  RA410.5.E43 2009
  338.4'73621—dc22   2009000907

9 8 7 6 5 4 3 2 1
The paper used in this publication meets minimum requirements of the American National
Standard for Information Sciences–Permanence of Paper for Printed Library Materials: ANSI
Z39.48-1992.

Typeset in Adobe Garamond

Composition by Circle Graphics, Inc.
Columbia, Maryland

Printed by Versa Press
East Peoria, Illinois

Center for Global Development

The Center for Global Development is an independent, nonprofit policy research organization dedicated to reducing global poverty and inequality and to making globalization work for the poor. Through a combination of research and strategic outreach, the Center actively engages policymakers and the public to influence the policies of the United States, other rich countries, and such institutions as the World Bank, the IMF, and the World Trade Organization to improve the economic and social development prospects in poor countries. The Center's Board of Directors bears overall responsibility for the Center and includes distinguished leaders of nongovernmental organizations, former officials, business executives, and some of the world's leading scholars of development. The Center receives advice on its research and policy programs from the Board and from an Advisory Committee that comprises respected development specialists and advocates.

The Center's president works with the Board, the Advisory Committee, and the Center's senior staff in setting the research and program priorities and approves all formal publications. The Center is supported by an initial significant financial contribution from Edward W. Scott Jr. and by funding from philanthropic foundations and other organizations.

Contents

Preface

For decades, governments in developing countries and the donors that support them have engaged in a "command-and-control" approach in the health sector: providing funding or in-kind resources for training, infrastructure, medicines, and other supplies and generating norms about what health workers should do (here are the inputs; use them this way).

While this approach has contributed to many improvements in health, and while dedicated individuals throughout the world are hard at work providing care, close observers of the sector have had a lingering sense that far more could be achieved—even within the limits of current health spending—if health workers showed up to work on time (or at all), if expectant mothers were better motivated to show up for pre-natal care, and if the churches and nongovernmental groups that manage rural health clinics were somehow more efficient. Frustration with the limits of the command-and-control input-based approach has grown as progress in child and maternal health has stalled in the poorest countries and as health systems in many countries have turned out to be unequal to the task of dealing with HIV/AIDS and drug-resistant TB.

In response came some controversial experiments. Instead of focusing exclusively on inputs and guidelines, several nongovernmental organizations, governments, and donors introduced payments linked to measured performance for health care providers and payments for mothers and other users of health services just for showing up.

In the spirit of CGD's signature "ideas to action" approach, Ruth Levine, a senior fellow and head of the Global Health Policy Program at the Center, and Rena Eichler, one of the pioneers in designing "pay-for-performance" programs in developing countries, document many of those experiences, on both the supply (provider) and demand (patient) sides. They acknowledge the risks associated with introducing explicit incentives and suggest ways to mitigate those risks. In the end, they recommend that donors pay far more attention to the potential of incentive payments—because they have real-world benefits when done right.

Understanding the promise and pitfalls of performance incentives fits squarely into the Center for Global Development's broader contributions to improvements in the effectiveness of development assistance. By bringing innovations to light, and providing policy guidance based on real-world experience, Eichler, Levine, and the contributors to this book highlight an alternative way for donors to support accelerated health improvements while inducing enduring changes in the way health care is financed, provided, and used. The authors do a great service by bringing together in one volume a discussion of incentives on the supply and demand sides and by tapping into knowledge from the United States and the United Kingdom. Seeing the growing interest in the application of performance incentives, I expect that this book will be a valuable resource for many years to come.

Nancy Birdsall
President
Center for Global Development
Washington, D.C.

Acknowledgments

The project that resulted in this book benefited from the involvement of many. We would like first to acknowledge the pioneers who designed and implemented performance-based incentive programs in developing countries. Their leadership and willingness to take the risk to deviate from "business as usual" are an inspiration; their willingness to share their experiences with a wider public is an act of generosity. Evidence from Afghanistan and Haiti inspires us all to believe that poor women and children can access essential maternal and child health services in the most challenged environments. Rwanda shows how committed national leaders can combine the best features of donor-funded pilots to create a national model that can be expanded to scale. Programs in Latin America and elsewhere that target the poorest by conditioning income supplements on the use of essential services teach us that motivating the poor with performance incentives can result in improvements in child health and nutrition. Innovations that have arisen from the "bottom up" in tuberculosis control programs, including incentives for both patients and health workers, have increased the likelihood that TB cases will be detected and cured.

We are deeply grateful to the members of the Center for Global Development's Performance-Based Incentives Working Group, who brought their expertise and passion to define the group's mandate and identify lessons and cases that showcase the best of existing knowledge. (See the profiles of working group members at the beginning of this book.) Composed of practitioners, policymakers, academics, and funders, this working group brought a wide spectrum of perspectives and experiences together. Our discussions about how to support the introduction of effective and appropriate incentives and how to understand and avoid problematic side effects produced the rich treatment of the issues covered in this volume. Contributing time and effort as committed volunteers, group members actively participated in meetings with a healthy dose of debate and contributed to and commented on countless drafts.

We would like to thank all the writers of cases for contributing the backbone of this book—the real-world cases that teach us what is possible and the lessons learned along the way. They present as concise a picture as possible of complex schemes and evidence of their impact.

Many reviewers helped us to present performance-based incentives in a manner understandable to broad audiences. George Schieber helped us to place the discussion of performance incentives within the policy discussions about health financing. Ricardo Bitran, Michael Clemens, Charles Griffin, April Harding, Marty Makinen, Mead Over, and Bill Savedoff provided valuable comments on specific case write-ups. All remaining errors are, of course, the responsibility of the authors and editors.

Our Center for Global Development colleagues have contributed constructive suggestions and provided support for this ambitious endeavor. In particular, sincere thanks are due to CGD President Nancy Birdsall and Vice President for Communications and Policy Lawrence MacDonald. Excellent research and organizational support was provided by Jessica Gottlieb, Danielle Kuczynski, and Scott Kniaz; we thank them very much for their dedication to this project.

We are grateful to the Bill & Melinda Gates Foundation for financial support and intellectual engagement in the working group process.

Abbreviations

ADB	Asian Development Bank
BTC	Belgian Technical Cooperation
CCT	Conditional cash transfer
CGD	Center for Global Development
DOT	Directly observed treatment
DOTS	Directly observed treatment, therapy short course
DTP	Diphtheria, tetanus, pertussis
EC	European Commission
ESIF	Emergency Social Investment Fund
FA	Familias en Acción, Colombia
FFSDP	Fully functional service delivery point
GAVI	Global Alliance for Vaccines and Immunization
HEDIS	Healthcare Effectiveness Data and Information Set
HIV/AIDS	Human immunodeficiency virus/acquired immunodeficiency syndrome
HMIS	Health Management Information System
IDB	Inter-American Development Bank
IFPRI	International Food Policy Research Institute
IHE	Institut Haitien de l'Enfance

IIHMR	Indian Institute of Health Management and Research
MDG	Millennium Development Goals
ISDP	Institutional service delivery point
MoPH-SM	Ministry of Public Health strengthening mechanism
NGO	Nongovernmental organization
ORT	Oral rehydration therapy
PAHO	Pan American Health Organization
PATH	Poverty Alleviation through Health and Education, Jamaica
PBI	Performance-based incentive
PBF	Performance-based financing
PEPFAR	President's Emergency Plan for AIDS Relief
PMTCT	Preventing mother-to-child transmission
PNFP	Private not-for-profit
PPD	purified protein derivative
PRAF	Programa de Asignación Familiar (Family Allowance Program), Honduras
REACH	Rural Expansion of Afghanistan's Community Based Healthcare
RPM Plus	Rational Pharmaceutical Management Plus
RPS	Red de Protección Social, Nicaragua
SILAIS	Local System of Integrated Health Care
TB	Tuberculosis
UNDP	United National Development Programme
UNICEF	United Nations Children's Fund
USAID	U.S. Agency for International Development
VCT	Voluntary counseling and testing
WHO	World Health Organization

Working Group Members

Led by Ruth Levine, the Performance-Based Incentives Working Group comprised twenty-six individuals with expertise in institutional and household economics, health finance and management, quality of care, and program implementation from throughout the world. The working group included the following members, who served in their individual capacity:

Carola Alvarez, a principal education and safety nets specialist at the Inter-American Development Bank (IDB), is concerned primarily with poverty and inequality, safety nets, and the economics of education. With work spanning empirical research, policy analysis, and implementation of best practices, she has focused on connecting lessons from implementation with empirical research. Alvarez has worked extensively in developing rigorous impact evaluation and providing technical assistance to the ministries of education of El Salvador and the Dominican Republic, the Oportunidades cash transfer program in Mexico, and the Programa de Asignación Familiar (PRAF) in Honduras. She has been task manager for IDB's loans to Mexico's Oportunidades program for the past five years.

Paul Auxila is a specialist in implementation strategies with a history of devising and managing major health programs that exceed expectations. A member of the Management Sciences for Health corporate senior management team and an industrial engineer with concentration in management engineering and systems design, he has been active in the field of international health management and development for the last twenty-six years. He is fluent in six languages and has worked extensively in more than thirty countries with both public and private sector colleagues and counterparts in the highest levels of government, academia, management, health services provision, and community work. Auxila is currently a Management Sciences for Health vice president and chief of party of the U.S. Agency for International Development (USAID) bilateral health project in Haiti.

Leslie Castro works with the Millennium Development Goals (MDG) Coordination and Territorialization Unit at the United Nations, which aims to strengthen the coherence of United Nations interagency efforts at the local level to achieve the MDG. She has extensive experience with the Ministry of the Family in Nicaragua, where she served as general director of programs and projects, overseeing three major World Bank programs: Red de Protección Social, Programa de Atención Integral a la Niñez, and the Attention to Crisis component. Before this, she served as director of the Red de Protección Social program as well as operations manager and technical manager, spending several years with this program. Castro holds two master's degrees, in sociology and in cooperation and development, both from Catholic University of Louvain-La-Neuve.

Karen Cavanaugh, health systems management analyst in the USAID's Bureau for Global Health, has twenty-two years of experience in designing, directing, and evaluating projects, programs, and organizations to improve health and mitigate poverty for people in Asia, Africa, the Middle East, Latin America, and the Caribbean. A member of the Global Alliance for Vaccines and Immunization (GAVI) health system strengthening task team, she oversees USAID's five-year $125 million Health Systems 20/20 project to strengthen health finance, governance, and operations worldwide and is engaged in creation of the new health systems action network. She is a member of the World Health Organization's steering committee on national health accounts.

David Cutler is Otto Eckstein Professor of Applied Economics in the faculty of arts and sciences and dean for social sciences at Harvard University. He served on the Council of Economic Advisors and the National Economic Council during the Clinton administration. Formerly with the National Institutes of Health and the National Academy of Sciences, Cutler is a research associate at the National Bureau of Economic Research and a member of the Institute of Medicine. He is the author of *Your Money or Your Life: Strong Medicine for America's Health Care System.*

Rena Eichler, president of Broad Branch Associates, concentrates on the application of incentives to improve health system performance. An economist with fifteen years of experience in the health sector working on national and local level policy development, implementation, and evaluation in Africa, Latin America and the Caribbean, Asia, the Middle East, and Eastern Europe, she develops projects and leads teams that provide technical assistance and conduct applied research. Eichler served as technical lead for the Performance-Based Incentives Working Group and as technical advisor to the interagency working group on results-based financing. As a partner on the USAID Health Systems 20/20 project, Eichler leads the global work program on pay for performance. She provides technical support to the World Bank on implementing the results-based financing strategy and has supported results-based financing activities for the government of Norway. She is engaged with the Brookings Institution in a program to examine performance-based aid in health. She was formerly employed by Harvard University, the U.S. Agency for Health Care Policy and Research, Management Sciences for Health, and the World Bank and has consulted for a wide range of development organizations.

Maha El-Adawy is the policy adviser for health in the United Nations Development Programme (UNDP). A medical doctor by background, she was program officer for reproductive health and reproductive rights in the Ford Foundation Office for the Middle East and North Africa before joining UNDP. She also worked with the European Union, USAID, and the World Bank on health sector reforms, consulted for the United Nations Children's Fund on child health issues, nutrition, and communication for behavioral change, and worked with several nongovernmental organizations. She cofounded an association to raise awareness about HIV/AIDS and to reduce related stigma in low-prevalence countries. A member of the International Union of Scientific Studies on Population, El-Adawy has lectured at Cairo University and published in the field of international population and health policy.

Luis Fernando Rolim Sampaio, a medical doctor specializing in hospital management who also holds a master's degree in public health, has worked as a policymaker since 1993, with lead positions at the municipal, state, and national levels in Brazil, including national director of primary health care. He helped to develop the Core Competencies of Primary Health tool for the Brazilian health system and represented the Brazilian Ministry of Health in the primary health care section of EUROSOCIAL. Sampaio participated in projects with the United Nations Educational, Scientific, and Cultural Organization (primary health care), Pan American Health Organization (family health), and the World Bank (Strengthen Family Health in Brazil). He now works at the University of Toronto, Canada.

Thomas Foels, a graduate of the University of Rochester School of Medicine and Dentistry and the Tulane University School of Public Health and Tropical Medicine,

established and managed two large medical group practices in western New York
and practiced clinical medicine at these sites for nearly sixteen years. He joined
Independent Health, the region's largest health maintenance insurer, as director of
practice management in 1994 and currently serves as medical director. Foels provides medical leadership in the design, development, and implementation of care
management, quality management, clinical policy, and utilization management.

Mark Gersovitz is professor in the Department of Economics at the Johns
Hopkins University. He specializes in development economics and has been
working on marrying economics and epidemiology. He also continues long-
standing interests in saving behavior and capital markets especially when willingness to repay is a constraint, agriculture, public finance, and international
commodity markets. He has been a consultant to the World Bank, the International Monetary Fund, and the UNDP and served as editor of the *World Bank
Research Observer* and the *World Bank Economic Review.*

Paul Gertler is a professor of economics and health services finance and faculty
director for the graduate program at the University of California, Berkeley. A faculty
research associate for the National Bureau of Economic Research, Gertler has
written extensively on health financing in developing countries for various publications and institutions, including the Pan American Health Organization and the
RAND Corporation, where he was a senior economist for eight years. Among other
honors, he received the Kenneth Arrow Award for Economics in 1996.

Amanda Glassman, a health financing specialist with more than fifteen years
of experience in health and social protection financing issues in Latin America
and elsewhere in the developing world, is lead health specialist at the Inter-
American Development Bank and a nonresident fellow at the Brookings Institution.
Before her current position, Glassman was deputy director of the Global Health
Financing Initiative at Brookings and carried out policy research on aid effectiveness in the health sector in lower-income countries. Before joining Brookings,
Glassman designed, supervised, and evaluated health and social protection loans
at the Inter-American Development Bank. Glassman holds a master of science
degree from the Harvard School of Public Health, has published on health
finance and policy topics, and is coauthor of *The Health of Women in Latin
America and the Caribbean* (World Bank 2001).

Markus Goldstein, a development economist with experience working in
Sub-Saharan Africa, East Asia, and South Asia, is currently with the Africa Region
of the World Bank, where he works as a senior economist on poverty and gender
issues. His research interests include HIV/AIDS, intrahousehold allocation, risk,
poverty measurement, public services, and land tenure. Before coming to the World

Bank, Goldstein taught at the London School of Economics and the University of Ghana, Legon. Author of several of articles and books on development issues, most recently he coedited the volume *Are You Being Served? New Tools for Measuring Service Delivery* (World Bank 2007).

Davidson Gwatkin serves as an adviser on health and poverty to the World Bank, United Nations Children's Fund, and other agencies. From 2000 to 2003, he was the World Bank's principal health and poverty specialist. Before joining the World Bank, he directed the International Health Policy Programs, a cooperative effort among two American foundations, the World Bank, and the World Health Organization to strengthen health policy research capacity in Africa and Asia. Gwatkin had previously been with the Ford Foundation in New Delhi, New York, and Lagos and with the Overseas Development Council in Washington.

Akramul Islam, currently program coordinator for tuberculosis (TB), malaria, and HIV/AIDS, Bangladesh Rural Advancement Committee Health Programme, has more than twenty years of experience working on TB in Bangladesh. Since 2005, he has held a faculty position at the School of Public Health at BRAC University, and in 2005 he was nominated for the Global Development Award 2000 by the World Bank in the category of environment and social sustainability for his research paper "Tuberculosis Control by Community Health Workers in Bangladesh: Is This More Cost-Effective?" Islam holds a doctorate of philosophy from Tokyo University in Japan, a master's degree in primary health care management from Mahidol University in Thailand, and a master of science degree from Bangladesh.

Daniel Kress is deputy director for policy and finance with the Global Health Delivery Team at the Bill and Melinda Gates Foundation in Seattle, Washington. Before joining the foundation, he worked at the World Bank as senior health economist in the Middle East and North Africa Region, and before that, he worked at Abt Associates on a variety of health care financing and health reform projects. As project director for the Sustainability and Financing of Immunizations Project, funded by the Children's Vaccine Program at Program on Appropriate Technologies in Health, he participated in a number of GAVI financing task force assignments and activities. Coauthor of a chapter for the Disease Control Priorities Project, Kress received his doctorate in economics from the University of North Carolina at Chapel Hill.

Kenneth Leonard is an assistant professor at the University of Maryland and a faculty associate at the Maryland Population Research Council. His research has focused on the delivery of key public services to rural populations in developing countries, specifically the delivery of curative health services, examining both supply and demand. Leonard has conducted research in Cameroon, Gabon, Kenya,

Tanzania, Ethiopia, and Uganda, and his work is published in economics journals (such as *Econometrica* and the *Journal of Economics Perspectives*), development journals (such as the *Journal of Development Economics*), and health economics journals (such as the *Journal of Health Economics, Social Science and Medicine,* and *Health Affairs*).

Ruth Levine, vice president for Programs and Operations at the Center for Global Development (CGD), is a health economist with more than fifteen years of experience working on health and family planning financing issues in East Africa, Latin America, the Middle East, and South Asia. Before joining the CGD, Levine designed, supervised, and evaluated health sector loans at the World Bank and the Inter-American Development Bank. From 1997 to 1999 she served as adviser on the social sectors in the Office of the Executive Vice President of the Inter-American Development Bank. Levine is the coauthor of *The Health of Women in Latin America and the Caribbean* (World Bank 2001) and *Millions Saved: Proven Successes in Global Health* (Center for Global Development 2004).

Philip Musgrove is a deputy editor of *Health Affairs,* the journal of health policy published by Project HOPE. Until his retirement in 2002, Musgrove served in a variety of capacities with the World Bank, the Pan American Health Organization, and the World Health Organization. He has worked on health reform projects in Argentina, Brazil, Chile, and Colombia as well as on a variety of issues in health economics, financing, equity, and nutrition. Widely published and author of more than fifty articles in economics and health journals and contributor to twenty books, Musgrove is adjunct professor in the School of Advanced International Studies, Johns Hopkins University, and has taught at George Washington University, American University, and the University of Florida.

Natasha Palmer has a master's degree in health policy and finance from the London School of Hygiene and Tropical Medicine, where she also completed her doctorate of philosophy. Since 1997, she has worked on health financing and contracting. She is a lecturer in health economics at the London School of Hygiene and Tropical Medicine, where she is affiliated with the Health Economics and Finance Programme.

John W. Peabody is medical director and senior vice president for Sg2, where he leads the Clinical Intelligence Programs, focusing on research development and program enhancement for the global health care market. Peabody is also a professor at the University of California, where he has been on the faculty since 1995 as the deputy director of the Institute for Global Health, part of the university-wide Global Health Sciences Program. He holds a rare joint appointment at University of California, San Francisco, in the Department of Epidemiology and Biostatistics and the Department of Medicine and at University of California, Los Angeles, in the Department of Health Services in the School of Public Health.

Miriam Schneidman, a senior health specialist at the World Bank, has more than twenty-five years of experience in health and human development issues in Africa and Latin America. Most recently, she was named coordinator of the Africa Regional TB Team at the World Bank, where she is leading an effort to scale up support for TB control in the region. With degrees in economics from the University of Maryland and in public health from Johns Hopkins University, Schneidman has written on vulnerable youth, demographic issues, community financing of health care, health problems of women, and HIV/AIDS. She is coauthor of *The Health of Women in Latin America and the Caribbean* (World Bank 2001).

Robert Soeters is a managing consultant at Verdonck, Klooster and Associates in the Netherlands. Before this, he was a senior development manager and business consultant at the same firm. With degrees from the Universiteit van Amsterdam, Small Business Haarlem, and Jacobus College, Soeters specializes in telecommunications, customer contact, new ways of communication and collaboration, mobility, and networking.

Sally Theobald is a senior lecturer in social science and international health at the Liverpool School of Tropical Medicine, United Kingdom. With a doctorate in gender, health, and development from the University of East Anglia, she works on gender equity and international health. Theobald has worked collaboratively on qualitative research projects on gender equity, HIV, TB, sexual and reproductive health, and health systems in Thailand, South Africa, Burkina Faso, Malawi, and Kenya.

Kevin Volpp, whose research focuses on the impact of financial and organizational incentives on health outcomes, has been working to use insights from behavioral economics to improve health behaviors. In several federally and privately funded randomized controlled trials, he has been testing the effectiveness of different incentive designs for reducing smoking, obesity, and failure to complete treatment. Recipient of the Presidential Early Career Award for Scientists and Engineers, the Outstanding Junior Investigator of the Year Award from the Society of General Internal Medicine, the John Thompson Prize from the Association of University Programs in Health Administration, and the Alice S. Hersh New Investigator Award from AcademyHealth, Volpp is director of the Center for Health Incentives at the Leonard Davis Institute, serves on the faculty of the University of Pennsylvania School of Medicine and the Wharton School, and is a board-certified internist and staff physician at the Philadelphia Veterans Affairs Medical Center.

Diana E. C. Weil, coordinator of policy and strategy for the Stop TB Department of the World Health Organization, has twenty years of experience in global public health policy analysis, program support, and disease control strategy development. Working with the World Health Organization, the Pan American Health Organization, and the World Bank, she has conducted analyses on the impact of development policies on health, the impact of health system reforms on disease control, the role for incentives and enablers in service delivery, anti-TB drug supply systems and markets, and priorities in operational research. Weil has served on numerous interagency panels and committees to devise innovative solutions in drug supply, health systems delivery and financing, and TB care and control.

PART ONE

More Health for the Money

1

Money into Health

Imagine a health clinic in a rural district in a poor country, far from the gatherings of global health headliners in Geneva, Washington, and Seattle. The staff working there—one doctor, two nurses, and a handful of community health workers—make an effort to respond when patients come in with health complaints. But medicines and equipment are in short supply, the building is in disrepair, and salaries are barely above subsistence levels. Those who fund the clinic's activities—perhaps the government, perhaps a nongovernmental organization (NGO) with headquarters in a distant city—ask few questions about how many patients are being served and whether health conditions are improving, although they require invoices accounting for all funds spent. Staff members struggle to feel motivated in the face of their daily challenges. They know that many of the poorest members of the community find it difficult to obtain the antenatal care and other basic services or treatments they need, but the health team rarely has the wherewithal to organize community health outreach efforts or to follow up on patients who might be failing to receive treatment for tuberculosis (TB) or AIDS.

Now, imagine that something changes. The young doctor, who is also the clinic manager, is told by his supervisor in the Ministry of Health or the NGO that the clinic budget will be increased by 10 percent if 20 percent more children in the community are vaccinated and if the number of TB patients completing a full course of treatment increases by 30 percent. Other changes also are introduced. Mothers in the community's poorest households receive modest monthly stipends if they can show that their children's vaccinations are up-to-date and that the children are being weighed and measured regularly at the local clinic. Health workers are directed to offer food packets to TB and AIDS patients each time they come in to obtain medicine.

What Will Happen and Why?

What will happen and why are questions worth answering and worth answering soon. The international community now devotes unprecedented resources and attention in an effort to attain ambitious goals to improve health in developing countries. In recent years, many billions of dollars have been pledged to prevent childhood death and disease through immunization and to treat and care for people affected by AIDS, malaria, and TB. Increasingly, donor agencies and philanthropists are recognizing that significant sums also are merited to reinforce maternal and child health interventions, and some global health leaders are urging new responses to the rapidly emerging threats of diabetes, tobacco-related ailments, and other chronic diseases in low- and middle-income countries. With national and provincial governments in developing countries joining with donors to devote ever-larger amounts to health services, whether those resources will improve health hinges on what is happening in those far-away clinics and households. And what is happening in those clinics and households has much to do with what influences the motivation and behavior of individual health workers, patients, and parents.

At the highest level, the focus has been on amounts of money raised for high-visibility health problems. A large share of the new donor funding is being provided through channels earmarked for specific diseases or interventions. The GAVI Alliance (formerly the Global Alliance for Vaccines and Immunization) provides grant funding to seventy-three low-income countries to buy vaccines and to improve the delivery of childhood immunization services. As of August 2008, it had approved some $4.1 billion for the period from 2000 to 2015.[1] As of February 2008, the Global Fund to Fight AIDS, Tuberculosis, and Malaria had approved more than $10 billion for health programs in 136 countries, and the sums may rise to as much as $8 billion per year through 2010.[2] The U.S. Presi-

---

1. See GAVI website, www.gavialliance.org/performance/commitments/index.php [October 2008].
2. See www.theglobalfund.org [October 2008].

dent's Emergency Plan for AIDS Relief plans to spend more than $60 billion over ten years on AIDS prevention, care, and treatment programs, focusing on fifteen countries. The U.S. President's Malaria Initiative, launched in June 2005, designs and implements malaria control programs in fifteen target countries. Its funding is expected to increase to $500 million in 2010.[3] The governments of Norway and the United Kingdom are backing ambitious plans for developing health systems in Africa, with a particular focus on reducing maternal and child mortality.

In an earlier era, funding for international health programs tended to be directed toward construction, training, and efforts to strengthen supply chains of the public sector and the health results were assumed to follow. Now the majority of donor monies are targeted more directly—for example, to reducing the number of deaths due to vaccine-preventable diseases, TB, malaria, and AIDS. The means are specific and, in concept, measurable: the proportion of babies and children immunized, the detection and effective treatment of TB among susceptible populations, the number of children and pregnant women who use insecticide-treated bed nets to protect against malaria-transmitting mosquitoes, the number of people with AIDS who are receiving and adhering to antiretroviral medicines, and the number of pregnant women who receive good antenatal care and deliver their babies under healthful conditions. Each of these indicators and many others have been embraced by results-oriented governments and donors. In very real ways, they represent what taxpayers in rich and poor countries alike think they are buying.

Achieving these objectives depends on the ability to translate good intentions and high-level financial commitments into a remarkably complex set of actions among the many individuals involved in any health system—from those who decide on the deployment of personnel and allocation of resources for buildings, drugs, and supplies to those who deliver and receive health services in the most remote locations in the poorest countries.

Arguably the most important actions, in fact, involve the delivery of services—the level farthest from the central sources of money, programmatic direction, and oversight. For example, if reducing maternal mortality depends on making sure that pregnant women receive timely prenatal care and deliver their babies with the assistance of trained attendants, then personnel in clinics must be motivated, empowered, and provided the resources to identify pregnant women in the community, to encourage them to come for checkups at appropriate moments, and to

3. See President's Malaria Initiative website, fact sheet, www.usaid.gov/press/factsheets/2006/fs060608.html [December 2008].

come to the health facility or seek assistance when labor commences. Much also depends on the behavior in households. The women and family members who affect their choices must themselves be motivated to seek care and to follow the guidance of health care providers about nutrition at home and the timing and type of care being sought. The same complex narrative can be constructed for virtually any of the health outcomes now at the top of the global and national agendas. At the end of the day, the new money, technologies, and hopes result in improved health only if those who are seeking and providing services act in particular ways.

The Argument

This book addresses one set of approaches to using money and other material goods to affect the actions of those who are delivering and receiving health services. More specifically, it is about how to use particular types of incentives—those that reward or penalize specific types of results—to motivate health-related behaviors. Performance incentives are defined as the transfer of money or material goods conditional on taking a measurable action or achieving a predetermined performance target. In the conceptualization we use, performance incentives include those that operate at the level of the health facilities (or networks of facilities), the individual provider, the household decisionmakers, and the patients. In other words, we look at incentives on both the demand and the supply sides, at both individual and collective levels. In our framework, we do not include the conditional payments that donor agencies offer to national governments, such as additional grant monies if and when particular policy decisions are made. We look solely at the interface between provider and patient.

We make no claims that performance incentives are the only or always the best way to generate improvements in the delivery and use of health services. At the same time, we do argue—by applying concepts from economics and, significantly, by closely examining a broad set of real-world experiences (see box 1-1)—that this approach should be prominent on the menu of ways to use donor and national government money. In particular, we recommend that donor agencies seeking to support particular types of health outcomes actively consider performance incentives as a way to use earmarked (vertical) funding to foster improvements—a way simultaneously to strengthen systems and achieve measurable results.

Performance incentives warrant both optimism and systematic assessment. Optimism is warranted because material incentives are powerful; when incentives

Box 1-1. *Case Summaries*

    —*Latin America: Cash transfers to support better household decisions.* Poor households receive income transfers as long as they access preventive services and attend health education talks.

    —*United States: Orienting pay-for-performance to patients.* Patients receive payments if they use priority services or change health-related behaviors.

    —*Afghanistan: Paying NGOs for performance in a postconflict setting.* Performance-based incentives are contrasted with input-based payment in a postconflict state with poor health statistics.

    —*Haiti: Going to scale with a performance-incentive model.* Supply-side incentives are given, as progressively more nongovernmental organizations are paid based on reaching population-based performance targets.

    —*Rwanda: Performance-based financing in the public sector.* Three donor-financed pilots are scaled up into a national model that rewards increased use of basic health services and services for communicable diseases, including HIV/AIDS.

    —*Nicaragua: Combining demand- and supply-side incentives.* Monetary transfers to households are linked to service use, and financial incentives for health providers are tied to the achievement of performance targets.

    —*Worldwide: Incentives for tuberculosis diagnosis and treatment.* Incentive schemes are targeted at patients and providers to increase case detection and motivate continued adherence to treatment.

have been introduced, the improvements in key health indicators have been large and rapid and appear to have exceeded what would have occurred in the absence of the incentive. Based on an emerging base of evidence, performance incentives appear to be effective ways to achieve important health gains. The positive effects have been demonstrated when only a relatively modest sum was used as the reward (or penalty). This suggests that performance-based elements can be usefully combined with—rather than replace—overall increases in spending on salaries, medicines, supplies, and infrastructure and may be a particularly strategic way to use a portion of the new resources available for health.

Being on the watch for potential pitfalls, however, is as important as being willing to innovate. Precisely because incentives are powerful, they call for careful design and implementation as well as monitoring of both intended and unintended consequences. Caution is warranted, in fact, for several reasons. One is that rigorous evaluations have been rare so far, and the body of evidence about the impact of performance incentives—though stronger than for many other approaches taken in global health—is not yet conclusive. Another is that monetary incentives enable those with flexible financial resources—often public and private donor agencies—to impose their own priorities. Finally, there is a set of potential unintended negative consequences, from undermining the integrity of information systems to inducing imbalance in the types of services provided, that have the potential to weaken the apparent benefits of performance incentives.

Organization of the Book

This volume, prepared with input from an expert working group (see box 1-2), is intended for policymakers and practitioners in the health sector in developing countries. We particularly focus on those in the donor community who are seeking to use resources as effectively as possible, are aware of the need to address shortcomings in health system performance, and may be considering or have already committed to a results-oriented approach. In chapter 2, we discuss three persistent health challenges in developing countries, highlighting issues related to how providers and patients behave: low use of services, inefficient services, and poor quality of services.

In chapter 3, we summarize knowledge from published and gray literature about the use of performance incentives in wealthy, middle-income, and poor countries. Chapter 4 moves to the elements of good design and implementation: what to consider when trying to understand the existing incentive environment, define indicators, set the targets and rewards, measure and verify performance, and more. Recognizing that the story on performance incentives is still being written, chapter 5 sets forth a learning agenda and a framework for evaluation. If shared across those who are financing and implementing programs that involve

---

Box 1-2. *Working Group on Performance Incentives*

The Center for Global Development convened the Working Group on Performance-Based Incentives in February 2006 (see the list of working group members at the beginning of this book). The working group brought together experts in health systems, incentive programs, and evaluation to review the available evidence and arrive at shared conclusions about the potential to apply various types of performance incentives in the health sector in low- and middle-income countries. Its explicit goals were to bridge the gap between demand- and supply-side approaches and to draw practical, policy-relevant conclusions from available knowledge about pay-for-performance experiences in low, middle- and high-income countries. This book is a result of both the deliberations of the working group and a set of case studies commissioned to inform the group's work.

performance incentives, that framework could yield a major expansion in the body of evidence about what works, what does not, and why.

In the second part of the volume, we present a series of cases about particular types of incentives (conditional cash transfers), particular countries (Haiti, Nicaragua, Rwanda, and Afghanistan), and a particular disease (TB). The cases give a feel for how programs are being implemented and what results are emerging when incentives are introduced, on both the demand and the supply sides.

2

Problems to Solve

In the vast majority of low-income countries, health system performance is way off the mark. Many of the individuals who could benefit most from preventive and therapeutic health services do not receive them, and when they do, the quality of the services is low. The most obvious reason for the deficiencies is limited resources. On average, low-income countries—those with a gross national income of less than $1,095 in 2009 dollars—spend about 4.1 percent of gross domestic product from both public and private sources. At current levels of spending, even adjusting for differences in the cost of labor and other inputs across countries, it is impossible for basic services of acceptable quality to reach the majority of the population. Beyond this, a range of systemic shortcomings is evident: quality control and supervision are absent, supply chains are broken, the transfer and use of information are weak, managerial skills are in short supply in both public and private sectors, and the absolute number of health workers at virtually all levels is lower than optimal by technical standards.

These problems are not found everywhere, but they are more the norm than the exception. It is against this backdrop that the global health community is seeking to make significant progress in the fight against leading causes of death and disability. And it is within this context that an active search for tools and solutions is under way.

To solve a problem, one must identify it and understand its underlying causes. Here we highlight both a set of important problems and the reasons to believe—at least on conceptual grounds—that introducing financial and other material incentives can improve health sector performance.

Identifying the Problems

Health system problems in low- and middle-income countries are not subtle. Essential and particularly preventive health services are little used, quality of care is low, and delivery of services is woefully inefficient.

Underused Services

Preventive, diagnostic, and even curative services are underused, particularly by the poor. Take childhood immunization, for example, which is universally regarded as one of the most cost-effective interventions in preventing life-threatening illnesses such as measles and neonatal tetanus. Currently, 27 million infants worldwide do not receive all three doses of DTP (diphtheria, tetanus, pertussis) vaccine, an indicator of whether they are fully immunized with the basic childhood antigens. Furthermore, across virtually all countries vaccination of children is much greater in wealthier households than in poorer households. A review of data from forty-four demographic and health surveys revealed that the rich-to-poor ratio for full immunization is 57:40 in nine countries of the Americas, 67:34 in twenty-two Sub-Saharan African countries, and 64:30 in four South Asian countries (Gwatkin, Wagstaff, and Yazbeck 2005). The picture is similar for other interventions, including dehydration from diarrhea and complications during pregnancy and childbirth (see figure 2-1). In the aggregate, public resources disproportionately reach the more affluent rather than the less so. In a study of twenty-one poor countries, for example, 15 percent of government health expenditures, on average, benefited the poorest 20 percent of households, yet more than 25 percent benefited the richest 20 percent (Filmer 2003).

Expanding the number of health facilities and placing them closer to where people live have helped to overcome some of the barriers to access, but the problem of underuse of essential services remains a prominent feature in many parts of the world. Even where physical access is relatively good, public health systems in the lowest-income countries suffer from poor quality, lack of trust between providers and members of the community, and limited outreach to individuals who do not spontaneously come for care. The result is the delivery of babies without benefit of

Figure 2-1. *Use of Health Services, by Income Quintile*

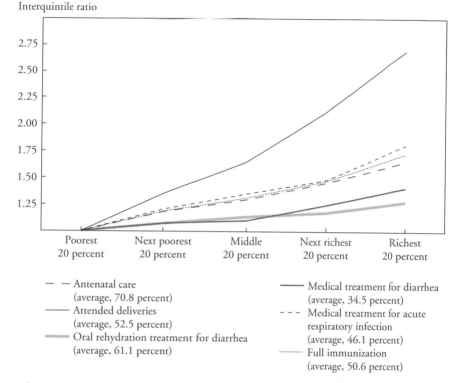

Interquintile ratio

— — Antenatal care
(average, 70.8 percent)
——— Attended deliveries
(average, 52.5 percent)
——— Oral rehydration treatment for diarrhea
(average, 61.1 percent)

——— Medical treatment for diarrhea
(average, 34.5 percent)
- - - Medical treatment for acute
respiratory infection
(average, 46.1 percent)
········ Full immunization
(average, 50.6 percent)

Source: Gwatkin, Wagstaff, and Yazbeck (2005).

prenatal care or skilled professionals during labor and the low use of cost-effective preventive and basic curative interventions.

Underuse is also evident in AIDS programs, where individuals may face the risk of social stigma if they use voluntary counseling and testing services. In Botswana, for example, use of voluntary counseling and testing services has been lower than anticipated despite the availability of free antiretroviral therapy for AIDS patients and widespread communications campaigns to motivate people to learn their HIV status.

In yet another form of underuse, many individuals do not adhere to a prescribed treatment for an infectious or chronic disease. The consequences are profound not only for individuals but also for society, in that drug resistance often emerges in the population. TB has drawn particular attention because of the potential for wider spread of the disease and the development of multidrug-resistant forms when patients do not complete the six-month course of treatment. An estimated 5 percent of new TB cases are resistant to multiple drugs, a reflection of systemic failure and discontinuity in treatment. Extensively drug-resistant TB, for which virtually no available drugs provide effective treatment, has also emerged. A similar issue involves first-line antiretroviral medications and the newer antimalarials.

Adherence to treatment regimes presents a challenge in managing non-communicable disease as well. With diabetes, for example, success depends on patients' changing their dietary behavior and taking insulin several times a day, indefinitely.

Low-Quality Care

Defined as "optimizing material inputs and practitioner skills to produce health" (Peabody and others 2006), quality is challenging to measure but widely regarded as seriously lacking in most developing-country health systems. Even if the observable dimensions, such as waiting times and provider courtesy, are adequate, the technical dimensions that patients cannot observe are not.

One way to get a sense of the magnitude of problems related to quality is to look at variation from technical norms of clinical practice. A seven-country study, based on direct observation of clinical practice, found that 75 percent of cases of common ailments, such as respiratory infection, were not adequately diagnosed, treated, or monitored. Inappropriate treatment, such as antibiotics for diarrheal disease, was offered in 61 percent of cases (Nolan and others 2001, cited in Peabody and others 2006). In a more recent study for the Disease Control Priorities Project, an international team used clinical vignettes to measure quality in China, El Salvador, India, Mexico, and the Philippines (Peabody and others 2006). The researchers found vast differences in quality among practitioners across all countries.

Low quality is related directly to the problem of underutilization. When patients who make the effort to seek care find that their condition does not improve with treatment, they may be less likely to seek care in the future or may turn to alternative—not necessarily more effective—services, such as traditional providers or home care.

Inefficient Delivery

Life (and health policy) would be far simpler if additional money and other material resources automatically translated into a healthier population. A host of studies have found that there is little relationship between health expenditures and infant and child mortality, controlling for other factors (summarized in Burnside and Dollar 1998; Musgrove 1996; Wagstaff and Claeson 2004). Other research has told a different story—that more spending on health systematically leads to improved health outcomes (including, among others, Gupta, Verhoeven, and Tiongson 2003; Baldacci, Guin-Siu, and de Mello 2002; Berger and Messer 2002; Anyanwu and Erhijakpor, n.d.). Virtually all who have looked at the question agree, however, that health outcomes depend on far more than the level of spending alone; the effectiveness of expenditures varies considerably depending on the characteristics and practices of health sector institutions.

Given how labor intensive health care is, the efficiency of the system depends crucially on the productivity and motivation of health workers, which is a function of their preservice preparation, the daily decisions they make on the job, as well as the environment in which they work. Systematic information about health worker productivity is limited, but several small-scale studies provide a troubling picture. Absenteeism averages around 50 percent, from a low of 19 percent in Papua New Guinea to a whopping 75 percent in Bangladesh (Lewis 2006). Workers fail to show up on time or leave early, particularly if they are engaged in other income-earning activities; sometimes they do not show up at all. Absenteeism is often seen in health systems characterized by explicit forms of corruption at the point of service delivery, such as siphoning off medicines for private gain and demanding side payments in exchange for services.

Recognizing the relationship between this problem and the others is important. When health workers have little motivation and are either absent or performing under their capacity, the results are manifested, at least in part, in low quality of service and potentially corrupt practices, such as side payments. All of these reinforce the problem of underuse. This vicious cycle is one in which poor health outcomes are almost inevitable.

It is tempting to conclude that most of the problems observed could be solved if the public sector had more money, either to provide or to purchase health services. It is certainly true that in low-income countries in particular the absolute levels of spending are below what could be expected to yield adequate health outcomes. But more resources alone are unlikely to be the sole answer. One study in Indonesia, for example, found that 60 percent of all perinatal deaths could be attributed to poor service delivery and only 37 percent to economic constraints (Supratikto and others 2002, cited in Peabody and others 2006).

Within the existing slim resource envelope, better services are possible. A study in Tanzania on the relative importance of ability and motivation in health worker performance found that clinicians do not always practice to the best of their ability (Leonard and Masatu 2005). The researchers observed the impact on health worker quality of being in an organization free to hire and fire staff and in which supervisors can set salaries. After controlling for the ability of the worker and the level of the facility, they found that clinicians working in such organizations demonstrated better performance.

When new funds are available—as they now are to provide care for individuals with HIV/AIDS, to combat malaria, and to increase immunization coverage— policymakers and program managers could think in whole new ways about how to use the new funds beyond a business-as-usual approach. The new resources are an opportunity to strengthen the delivery of health services by focusing on what the health system produces rather than what it consumes.

Using Performance Incentives

Translating funding into health entails thinking about forces that are invisible yet powerful: incentives that induce behavior associated with good or bad health outcomes. The behaviors that correspond to standard incentives are unlikely to produce the best outcomes, however. In the public sector, where managers and providers tend to be paid salaries based on seniority, the incentive structure often results in providers failing to exert significant effort to undertake patient outreach, to follow up to ensure adherence to medication regimes, to ensure that the logistics system runs smoothly, to use the knowledge acquired in training, or to go the extra mile in other ways. The problem of absenteeism described earlier is the most vivid example.

In the private sector, by contrast, providers tend to be paid per service and more for some types, such as curative services, than for others, such as preventive care and health education. Under these circumstances, the tendency may be to over-provide the more lucrative types of care and to underprovide the less profitable ones. For instance, overprescribing medication has been a chief complaint in the Indian private sector, where drug sales are a primary source of revenue (Bhat 1999). In both public and private sectors, conventional financing approaches provide few incentives to seek out hard-to-reach and hard-to-care-for individuals, who may themselves face major and competing demands on their resources and time.

Designing effective systemic interventions in health service delivery requires understanding who has to change behavior to improve outcomes. For the sake of (considerable) simplicity, let us say that four key actors make decisions relevant to health outcomes. One is the government or other financiers, which might include donors or private insurers. Another is the service manager, who might be the government official responsible at a local level or the manager of a nongovernmental clinic or network of health facilities. A third is the health care provider (again, public or private) who deals directly with patients. Last is the patient or the persons who make decisions on his or her behalf.

Relationships among these actors are complex, characterized simultaneously by two factors. First, different actors are privy to different types of information relevant to health care decisionmaking. Patients may know whether they are taking their medicine, but the provider and the financier may not. Providers may know whether they are doing everything possible to achieve a positive health outcome. The manager, the financier, and the patient may not. The financier is also in the dark about the quantity and quality of service. Health services are provided and received by a set of widely dispersed individuals, usually operating without on-the-spot supervision. No imaginable level of monitoring could overcome all of the asymmetries in information that characterize the health sector.

Second, different actors have different objectives and preferences. Financiers may wish to obtain the best possible health result for a fixed budget; managers may wish to achieve and maintain a good institutional reputation as a way to expand market share; providers may seek to earn as much money as possible, within some professional constraints, whether through direct service charges or side payments. Providers, managers, and financiers may all want the highest success rate of treatment across the population of patients, but some patients may value the near-term experience associated with unhealthful habits, such as tobacco use, more than the long-term benefits of healthful behaviors, such as exercise and good nutrition.

This is the principal-agent problem in health, where a principal wants an agent to provide or use a particular kind of service in a particular way to achieve the principal's objectives—for example, improved health status or lower cost per case treated. The lack of ability to monitor, against the background of competing preferences and objectives of agents, creates a problem for the principal that is not easily solved.

The original formulation of the principal-agent problem in health service delivery, which grew out of the groundbreaking work of Nobel laureate Kenneth Arrow on the role of information in economic behavior (Arrow 1963), focused on the ways in which the physician is the agent of the patient (as principal). The patient has relatively little information about the efficacy of treatments or the skill of the provider, yet must count on the physician to act in the patient's best interests at all times. In reality, health care is characterized by multiple principals and multiple agents, the provider being the agent of the patient, the provider being the agent of the financier, or the patient being the agent of the financier.

From a public policy perspective, a government or donor agency financier (and sometimes a corporate or philanthropic financier) can be thought of as a principal with an interest in reducing inequities in the use of health services, promoting consumption of health services that reduce the incidence or severity of infectious diseases and other conditions that harm society, and ensuring efficient health spending. Toward these ends, both the current and the potential patients as well as the providers and the institutions that may employ them (such as nongovernmental organizations or clinic networks) are agents of this principal.

To achieve these objectives, given the asymmetries in information and divergent agent aims, the principal has few options. Strategies that depend on direction from a central authority are extremely unlikely to work. Not only is a central authority unable to know the specifics of a given case, but it also cannot monitor the multitude of provider-patient interactions and enforce norms about how to treat patients with particular conditions, for example. And it certainly cannot ensure that individuals who would benefit from particular kinds of preventive or other health services will make the effort to obtain them.

The classic solution is for the principal to introduce financial rewards and penalties to create incentives for the agent to adopt particular behaviors, with independent monitoring as a necessary adjunct. Incentive theory has been elucidated by Laffont and Martimort (2001), among others, and has given rise to a large number of applications. Most of these have taken the form of contracts, specifying the measurable performance targets, the penalties and rewards, and the method of monitoring. In some cases, the performance aims are vague and the bar is low, with penalties and rewards as simple as termination or continuation of the contract, as is the case for most employment contracts. We apply a narrower definition of performance-based incentives: *monetary payments or other material rewards that are provided on the condition that one or more indicators of performance change, that predetermined targets are met, or both.* Because it is impossible to specify every desired element of service delivery or behavior, and the most important intangibles of provider-patient interactions cannot be monitored at reasonable cost, contract design implies identifying proxy measures that both can be monitored and represent a constellation of good behaviors. Contract design also must guard against unintended consequences (see box 2-1).

Using their power as purchasers, governments (with or without donor support) and private insurers can use the way they pay for services to encourage patients, providers, and health system managers to behave in particular ways associated with

Box 2-1. *Unintended Consequences to Avoid: Displacement of Intrinsic Motivation and Gaming*

As the theory and application of incentives have developed, questions have been raised about whether material incentives displace or conflict with intrinsic motivation. In health service delivery, for example, health care workers may have a strong sense of professionalism, reinforced by peers and their own self-image, which encourages them to provide high-quality care. Incentives that provide rewards for following clinical protocols, for example, or for providing preventive services may be redundant and bring little or no change in practices or outcomes. Worse, an incentive program may reduce intrinsic motivation, so that the health care workers provide only the services for which they are explicitly rewarded and not those they might have provided under other circumstances. Worse still, an incentive program may convey a lack of trust on the part of the management or funder and lead to a reduction in quality. When intrinsic motivation is high and based in part on a relationship of trust between principal and agent, incentives can have a perverse effect on performance (for an in-depth treatment, see Ellingsen and Johannesson 2006). In designing incentives, care must be taken to understand patterns of intrinsic motivation and to ensure that incentives support high performers rather than reflect mistrust of workers.

The introduction of new incentives may tempt those who wish to game the system. Gaming can occur if providers or other agents adapt their behavior to respond to the letter but not the spirit of the contract, disconnecting the performance indicator from the range of behaviors for which it is thought to be a proxy. For example, a health care worker can game a contract that includes a target for well-child visits by providing only a subset of appropriate preventive and diagnostic services at each visit. Similarly, a clinic rewarded on the basis of the share of patients from low-income households could achieve a high score by discouraging high-income patients and lowering the overall level of use. In both cases, the agent subverts the intention of the principal to his or her advantage, while precisely following the rules of the game. It is in the design (and revision) of the contract terms that opportunities for gaming can be minimized.

better health outcomes. For patients, this may mean providing cash or offering food or other material incentives to encourage them to obtain services they otherwise would not, to adhere to a treatment regime, or to engage in healthful behaviors, such as exercise or smoking cessation. The transfers can be seen both as incentives and as enablers, permitting patients to pay for transport or other indirect costs that might otherwise serve as a barrier to care. For providers, it may mean providing salary increments or fee-for-service bonuses for particular types of services or for improved quality of care, such as following treatment guidelines. For managers, it may mean conditioning institutional payments under contracts on the achievement of particular targets for service delivery, adherence to quality-related protocols, or even changes in population health.

Conclusions

Performance incentives have intuitive appeal. They have the potential to partially solve one or more of the problems that arise when payment for health care is disconnected from results and thus encourage perverse behaviors. Better outcomes aside, they permit financiers to move away from the micromanagement associated with accounting for and examining the use of each input and toward a more hands-off approach where the desired results are what is counted. Perhaps more significant, well-designed performance incentives may be an important way to invest in the core capabilities of those who are making the choices that are the strongest determinants of health outcomes. On the demand side, when mothers are paid a monthly stipend on the condition that they take their child for well-child services and growth monitoring, the payments can contribute to the accrual of human capital over the long term. On the provider side, when networks of facilities are paid on the basis of results, rather than on periodic budgets, they may establish the well-functioning management information, personnel, logistics, and other systems that will have long-term benefits. The question, then, is not whether performance incentives might be a useful tool to improve health and health systems. The promise is clear. But under what conditions, and how?

References

Anyanwu, John C., and Andrew E. O. Erhijakpor. n.d. "Health Expenditures and Health Outcomes in Africa." Unpublished paper. Washington: World Bank.

Arrow, Kenneth. 1963. "Uncertainty and the Welfare Economics of Medical Care." *American Economic Review* 53 (5) (December): 941–43.

Baldacci, Emanuele, Maria Teresa Guin-Siu, and Luiz de Mello. 2002. "More on the Effectiveness of Public Spending on Health Care and Education: A Covariance Structure Model." IMF Working Paper WP/02/90. Washington: International Monetary Fund.

Berger, Mark C., and Jodi Messer. 2002. "Public Financing of Health Expenditures, Insurance, and Health Outcomes." *Applied Economics* 34 (17): 2105–13.

Bhat, Ramesh. 1999. "Public-Private Partnerships in Health Sector: Issues and Prospects." Ahmendabad: Indian Institute of Management.

Burnside, Craig, and David Dollar. 1998. "Aid, the Incentive Regime, and Poverty Reduction." Macroeconomics and Growth Group Paper. Washington: World Bank.

Ellingsen, Tore, and Magnus Johannesson. 2006. "Pride and Prejudice: The Human Side of Incentive Theory." *American Economic Review* 98 (3): 990–1008.

Filmer, Deon. 2003. "The Incidence of Public Expenditures on Health and Education." Background Note for *World Development Report 2004: Making Services Work for Poor People.* Washington: World Bank.

Gupta, Sanjeev, Marijn Verhoeven, and Erwin Tiongson. 2003. "Public Spending on Health Care and the Poor." *Health Economics* 12 (8): 685–96.

Gwatkin, Davidson R., Adam Wagstaff, and Abdo S. Yazbeck, eds. 2005. *Reaching the Poor with Health Nutrition and Population Services.* Washington: World Bank.

Laffont, Jean-Jacques, and David Martimort. 2001. *The Theory of Incentives: The Principal-Agent Model.* Princeton University Press.

Leonard, Kenneth L., and Melkiory C. Masatu. 2005. "The Use of Direct Clinician Observation and Vignettes for Health Services Quality Evaluation in Developing Countries." *Social Science and Medicine* 61 (9): 1944–51.

Lewis, Maureen. 2006. "Tackling Health Care Corruption and Governance Woes in Developing Countries." CGD Brief. Washington: Center for Global Development.

Musgrove, Philip. 1996. "Public and Private Roles in Health: Theory and Financing Patterns." Discussion Paper 339. Washington: World Bank.

Nolan, Terry, Patria Angos, Antonio J. Cunha, Lulu Muhe, S. Quazi, E. A. Simoes, G. Tamburlini, M. Weber, and N. F. Pierce. 2001. "Quality of Hospital Care for Seriously Ill Children in Less-Developed Countries." *Lancet* 357 (9250): 106–10.

Peabody, John W., Mario M. Taguiwalo, David A. Robalino, and Julio Frenk. 2006. "Improving the Quality of Care in Developing Countries." In *Disease Control Priorities in Developing Countries,* 2d ed., edited by Dean T. Jamison and others. Washington: World Bank.

Supratikto, Gunawan, Meg E. Wirth, Emdang Achadi, Surekha Cohen, and Careine Ronsmans. 2002. "A District-Based Audit of the Causes and Circumstances of Maternal Deaths in South Kalimantan, Indonesia." *Bulletin of the World Health Organization* 80 (3): 228–34.

Wagstaff, Adam, and Miriam Claeson. 2004. *The Millennium Development Goals for Health: Rising to the Challenge.* Washington: World Bank.

3

Using Performance Incentives

When the goal is to reduce needless death and disease, and part of what is getting in the way is a misalignment between health goals and the real-world behaviors of individual patients, health workers, and those who influence them, it may be time to consider performance incentives (see box 3-1 for a description of the basic kinds of performance incentives). These can complement other interventions, such as providing training, revamping infrastructure, and improving the supply of drugs and other inputs. Here we look at how performance incentives can contribute to better health results, increased use of services, enhanced quality, and improved efficiency.

To identify the experiences to highlight in this book, we searched the published literature, consulted experts, and included regional and national cases with substantial documented evidence. The evidence discussed here and in the case summaries in part 2 relies on both evaluations conducted with varying degrees of rigor and other sources of information. It comes from qualitative surveys, baseline and endline statistics, contrasts between intervention and comparison groups, and routine program monitoring.

Demand-side interventions have tended to benefit from the most rigorous evaluations, partly because of the larger samples that are feasible with interventions at the household level. Evaluations of supply-side interventions in both developed

Box 3-1. *A Menu of Performance Incentives*

Performance incentives take a variety of forms and can be applied both to paying those who provide health services and those who use them. Performance incentives include:

On the supply side

Payments for achieving improvements in population health and/or health service coverage by district or municipality, or penalty for failing to meet targets

Payments for achieving service delivery targets at the level of the health care facility, or penalty for failing to meet targets

Payments for achieving service delivery targets by individual health workers, or penalty for failing to meet targets

Payments to facilities or individuals for incremental increases in a set of services: more appropriate for underutilized preventive care services than services with the potential of being excessively utilized ("supply induced demand")

On the demand side

Income support to poor households in which children obtain particular preventive health care services, such as immunization, and have good school enrollment and attendance records ("conditional cash transfers")

Cash payment, food support, or other goods to paients who take a particular health-related action, such as obtaining a screening test, adhering to treatment, or engaging in behavior modification programs that encourage smoking or drug cessation

and developing countries have used a diverse set of methods and, in general, have been methodologically less rigorous. Regardless of the methods, however, in most cases it is not possible to attribute improved results solely to the newly introduced incentive. For example, decreases in stunting associated with conditional cash transfer programs are attributable partly to increases in income that enable poor households to purchase food and partly to the incentive effect. Similarly, when the incentives have been provided to health care workers or managers, disentangling the impact of the incentive from that of other interventions introduced simultaneously is problematic. Whether expectations have been clearly communicated and monitored also can be a factor. Much of the available evidence suggests that performance incentives do have a positive impact, but it is also significant that the relative scarcity of negative results may be related to publication bias, which favors cases that show success over those that show little or no impact (see box 3-2 for an experiment in Uganda that showed little impact). In short, the base of evidence is far from perfect, but it is substantial enough to support the design of policy and program. Throughout this chapter, we take care when drawing inferences from the limited base of evidence, while at the same

Box 3-2. *Uganda: Can Performance Bonuses Improve the Delivery of Health Services?*

The government of Uganda was interested in knowing whether persistent low performance could be improved within the constraints of a limited budget. To answer this question, researchers from the World Bank, Makerere University Institute of Public Health, and the Uganda Ministry of Health undertook a rigorous field experiment to study the impacts of performance-based contracts between the government (as purchaser) and private not-for-profit (PNFP) health service providers.

Sixty-eight facilities from five districts participated. PNFPs account for about one-third of all health facilities in the country and about half of all health services provided. Participating facilities were randomly assigned to one of three study arms: two intervention groups (A and B) and a control group (C). Facilities in group C received a government grant restricted to the purchase of specific inputs and the delivery of specific services and defined outputs. Those in group B also received the grant, but were given freedom to spend funds without restriction. Those in group A were given freedom of allocation as well as a bonus payment if they achieved three self-selected targets of six: increases in outpatient visits, treatment of malaria in children, immunizations, antenatal visits, attended births, and uptake of family planning.

Collected in three survey waves, the study showed increasingly better performance for group A. Similar increases were seen in groups B and C. Statistical analyses of the average effect of performance bonuses revealed no significant difference across groups. In fact, for a few outcomes, group B performed better than the others.

The researchers offered three explanations. First, the bonuses were small: approximately 5 to 7 percent of operating revenue. Second, the contract was complicated, and putting the systems in place to manage it took time. Third, the scheme was offered for only two years, leaving facilities little time to respond to new incentives and demonstrate improved results.

Source: Lundberg, Marek, and Pariyo (2007).

time, realizing that decisions will be made even in the absence of rock-solid research, we highlight where the range of information seems to be pointing.

In considering performance incentives and results, we use two complementary lenses: the first focuses on health results for diseases or health interventions that are clear international priorities, while the second focuses on how performance incentives can strengthen health systems, which is increasingly being seen as an objective of donors and national governments. The disease-intervention lens presents evidence from specific case results for diseases such as tuberculosis, preventive care such as child immunizations, and priority services such as safe deliveries. The system lens looks at how performance incentives, instead of or along with more traditional solutions, can address the common problems of underuse, poor quality, and inefficiency.

Diseases and Interventions

Performance incentive schemes have been applied across a range of interventions, from time-limited services such as immunizations to chronic conditions such as diabetes and from preventive strategies such as prenatal care and growth monitoring to screening to detect cancer and hypertension. They have also been used to encourage people to be tested for infectious diseases such as tuberculosis (TB) or HIV/AIDS and to adhere to long treatment regimens.

When designing incentives, it is useful to draw lessons from other health conditions that have similar attributes. Figure 3-1 is a stylized and subjective attempt to categorize interventions based on duration and the intensity of behavioral changes required. Close to the origin, showing discrete time-limited interventions and minimal to no change in behavior, is the low-hanging fruit of performance

Figure 3-1. *Subjective Categorization of Health Interventions*

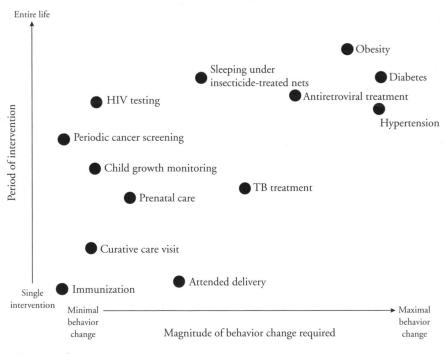

Source: Authors.

incentives. Included as examples are childhood immunizations, attended deliveries, curative care visits, child growth monitoring, and disease testing. The far right of the figure shows lifetime conditions, such as diabetes, hypertension, and addiction, for which effective management requires significant changes in daily behavior. Conditions such as tuberculosis, for which treatment is finite and behavioral changes are concentrated on medications and regular monitoring, show up somewhere in the middle.

Measurable Interventions

The best candidates for incentives appear to be services that require few if any behavioral changes, can be measured, and are offered for a limited time. Evidence from supply-side programs demonstrates that financial incentives are effective for immunization efforts. All of the examples of supply-side incentives in this book include immunization coverage targets; each case resulted in a measurable increase in rates for providers that were offered an incentive over either those that were not or the overall trend in the region.

In Haiti, for example, the increase among nongovernmental organizations (NGOs) in the performance payment scheme was, on average, between 13 and 24 percentage points higher than among other NGOs (see chapter 9). In Rwanda, the difference was nearly 10 percentage points (see chapter 10). Similarly, a study from the United States (Fairbrother and others 1999) demonstrated that paying bonuses to physicians increased immunization coverage much more rapidly than subsidizing vaccination fees or providing better feedback to physicians, by 25.3 percentage points over the other groups. The study cautions that because the scheme also improved documentation, some of the perceived impact may be attributable to data rather than to coverage.

Improving immunization coverage also has been tackled through conditional cash transfers (CCTs). A study of the impact of CCTs in Mexico and Nicaragua on groups not reached with the usual supply strategies—for example, children living farther from a health facility and having a mother with less than a primary school education—found a significant impact on immunization rates (Barham, Brenzel, and Maluccio 2007). The impact on immunization coverage of CCTs, however, has systematically been less than that of supply-side performance-based incentive programs, perhaps because the evidence on CCTs comes primarily from Latin America, where immunization coverage is relatively high, while the supply-side experiences are from settings where the baseline coverage rate was far lower.

Although somewhat more demanding than vaccination in terms of behavioral change, supply-side incentives have also been used to improve child nutrition.

One major cause of malnutrition in the developing world—diarrhea—was addressed with provider incentives to improve the use of oral rehydration therapy (ORT) in Bangladesh. Health workers charged with teaching mothers how to deal with diarrheal disease were rewarded on the basis of indicators such as the ability of mothers to prepare the ORT solution correctly. A pilot project showed positive results and was subsequently scaled up (Chowdhury 2001).

Increasing access to basic services is a priority when use is low and mortality and morbidity are high. In Rwanda after the genocide, for example, supply-side incentives were introduced (see chapter 10): where providers were paid in part on the basis of the number of curative care services provided, per capita consultations increased by 0.3 (from 0.22 to 0.55) versus only 0.1 (from 0.2 to 0.3) among the comparison group. However, documenting an increase in quantity is one thing. Determining the quality of diagnosis and treatment is much more challenging.

Several programs have also introduced supply-side incentives to increase the use of maternal health services. Improvement in attended deliveries appears possible in a relatively short period; increases in prenatal care, however, appear to take longer. In Rwanda, institutional deliveries increased from 12 to 23 percent in provinces with performance-based financing, versus 7 to 10 percent elsewhere (see chapter 10). In Haiti, NGOs that were paid based on performance were able to achieve an increase in attended deliveries of between 17 and 27 percentage points over their counterparts (see chapter 9). In Israel in the 1950s, a performance incentive increased attended deliveries among Bedouin women when mothers were entitled to maternity allowances—free hospitalization and a cash grant—if they gave birth in a hospital rather than at home or with a tribal midwife, as custom dictated. Initially the promise of cash was the strongest motivator, but over time, the benefits of Western medicine also provided an incentive (Shvarts and others 2003).

Supply-side performance incentives appear well suited to motivate screening for conditions that affect a large portion of the population. In the United States, they have been used to encourage pap smears, mammograms, and blood pressure screening (see box 3-3). In 2000, for example, the managed care plan Touchpoint offered monthly bonuses to physicians achieving improvements in services included in the National Committee for Quality Assurance's Healthcare Effectiveness Data and Information Set (HEDIS).[1] Its success—the third highest breast cancer

---

1. HEDIS is a tool used by more than 90 percent of America's health plans to measure performance on important dimensions of care and service. For more information, see web.ncqa.org/tabid/59/Default.aspx [October 2008].

Box 3-3. *United States: Lessons from the Supply Side*

Some estimates show that patients in America's complex health care system may receive as little as 55 percent of recommended care (McGlynn and others 2003). Pay for performance, begun in the private sector by large employers concerned about value for their spending, is therefore generating significant excitement as an option to improve quality of services (Kindig 2006). A 2001 report by the Institute of Medicine, *Crossing the Quality Chasm,* advocated a redesign of the entire system. Recent reforms now require centers that provide Medicare and Medicaid services to adopt pay for performance to address concerns about variability and quality of services (Rosenthal and Dudley 2007). These are substantial. Projected lifetime Medicare costs in Los Angeles, for example, are $84,000 greater than those in Seattle (Wenneberg and others 2007), and the cost of a mastectomy for breast cancer in one part of Pennsylvania is triple that in another (Guggenheim 2005).

As of 2005, approximately 157 initiatives covered more than 50 million enrollees in the United States (Sobrero and others 2006). The majority of pay-for-performance schemes—representing 80 percent of enrollees—have been with health maintenance organizations, primarily because evaluation is problematic in looser organizational forms such as preferred provider organizations (Rosenthal and others 2006; Gilmore and others 2007). Various independent organizations have also been established to encourage the use of pay for performance and participation in public reporting. Among them are Bridges to Excellence and Leapfrog Group.

Evaluating Pay for Performance
Rigorous evaluations have been sparse overall, and results have been mixed. The literature, however, is growing. Research identifies consensus on a number of common characteristics important in the design of pay for performance, including the magnitude of the incentive, the proportion of each provider's patients to whom the incentive scheme applies, and the costs of improving quality (Dudley 2005), as well as consideration of whether the incentive was used in the private or the public sector. Valuable findings from across settings—the influence of local factors (Trude and Au 2006; Felt-Lisk, Gimm, and Peterson 2007), the timing of incentives (Petersen and others 2006; Khan III and others 2006), and reward disparities (Rosenthal and others 2005; Lindenauer and others 2007) among them—also are emerging.

Pay for Performance Tomorrow
Three major policy issues surround pay-for-performance efforts in the United States: lack of guidance for purchasers on effective design, variation among payers on the clinical domains and quality measures to target, and concerns about escalating costs. Designing pay-for-performance schemes is complex and involves population-level factors (Kindig 2006), attitudes of physicians (Young and others 2007), the ability of organizations (Christianson, Knutson, and Mazze 2006) and systems to handle reforms, plus timing, organizational, and economic factors (Town and others 2004). The growing body of knowledge about how these schemes work will provide fuel for future designs.

screening rate in the country in 2004—is attributed to the competition stimulated among physicians and the implementation of an aggressive patient follow-up scheme. Other results indicate that incentives in combination with HEDIS measures also may have played a role in raising the rates of screening for breast cancer and cervical cancer (Baker and others 2004). Similar results can be seen across time. In a follow-up study of twenty-seven early adopters of performance incentives in the United States, Rosenthal and colleagues found that, since 2003, mammography and other screening indicators eventually were dropped from schemes because of consistently high success (Rosenthal and others 2007).

To increase rates of testing for HIV/AIDS and to motivate people to return to learn the results, people in Malawi were randomly assigned monetary incentives. Without incentives, demand was moderate at 39 percent. When a modest payment was offered, the response more than doubled (Thornton 2005). Monetary incentives may also help to overcome social stigma by enabling the perception that the reason for returning is to receive the money rather than to hear the test results.

Time-Limited Interventions

Many important health interventions occur for an extended but still finite period. These include child growth monitoring, prenatal and postnatal care, family planning, tuberculosis treatment, and sleeping under insecticide-treated bed nets to prevent malaria. What all these have in common is that they either imply repeated contacts with health providers (child growth monitoring, prenatal care, tuberculosis) or require changes in daily behaviors (sleeping under insecticide-treated bed nets, family planning).

Demand-side incentive programs have succeeded in improving child nutrition outcomes. Child growth monitoring is included in nearly all cash transfer programs, and most report positive results for nutritional outcomes. Stunting among girls decreased as much as 29 percentage points in Mexico, 5.5 points in Nicaragua, and 6.9 points in Colombia. The results are not unambiguous, however. The influence of the incentive is hard to separate from the effects of the cash transfer on the household food budget. Results from unconditional cash transfer programs also showed positive impacts on nutritional status (Agüero, Carter, and Woolard 2006). Programs need to be monitored for unintended consequences. In Brazil, for example, researchers attributed declines in nutritional status to a perception that benefits would be discontinued if the child showed improvement (Morris and others 2004).

The effect of supply-side incentives on the use of prenatal services appears to take longer than that of immunizations or attended deliveries. In Haiti, the lag was two years (see chapter 9). Interviews with stakeholders in Haiti suggest that service providers cannot immediately establish the systems needed to attract pregnant women to come in for care early and regularly. In Rwanda, early evidence showed no significant increase in prenatal care (see chapter 10).

In western Kenya, free antimalaria bed nets were given to pregnant women as incentives to increase enrollment at a prenatal clinic providing a range of services that included HIV testing. In the program area, use of prenatal care services increased by 117 percent and generated an 84 percent increase in the uptake of HIV testing services by women (Dupas 2005). The program makes it clear that incentives to improve one health behavior (in this case, prenatal care) can be designed to have spillover effects on other health outcomes (in this case, malaria prevention).

Conditional cash transfer programs that require pregnant women to receive prenatal care have shown improvements (see chapter 6). In Mexico's CCT program, poor families received monthly income transfers equivalent to between 20 and 30 percent of income if (among other conditions) pregnant women visited clinics to obtain prenatal care, nutritional supplements, and health education (Gertler 2004). Early rigorous evaluations of the program found that the number of women making their first prenatal care visit during their first trimester of pregnancy rather than in later stages increased by 8 percent (Sedlacek, Ilahi, and Gustafsson-Wright 2000).

Because incentives do alter behavior, designers need to ensure that the incentives do not result in unintended outcomes and must be exceptionally careful when determining how to link payments with reproductive health and family planning services. To this end, the U.S. government passed the Tiahrt Amendment, a law prohibiting the use of U.S. development assistance to introduce financial incentives to coerce people to limit family size or use contraceptives. In Haiti, in the spirit of encouraging voluntarism, providers were rewarded for having a full menu of modern contraceptives available in the first pilot year (see chapter 9). In later years, rewards were added for reducing the rate of discontinuation of contraceptive use by those who started to use the methods. This indicator was initially viewed as complying with the spirit of voluntarism, but was subsequently dropped in response to concerns that it was coercive or could be perceived to be so.

Incentives on the demand side can also run into complications. Demand-side programs can have perverse impacts on family size and the decision to use family planning. For example, CCT programs that base the size of the income transfer on household size may include apparent incentives for a household to have more children than it would have without an income support program. Programs in Colombia, Mexico, and Nicaragua were associated with decreases in fertility rates, but the program in Honduras, which applied a different incentive structure, saw an increase. One strategy that may not generate perverse effects is the requirement to attend health education talks about the benefits of family planning and effective contraception.

One time-limited and measurable intervention, the treatment of tuberculosis, appears to be a good candidate for performance incentive schemes. Many TB control programs incorporate incentives such as direct payment, food packages or vouchers, and transportation assistance to support access to World Health Organization–approved treatment and enable increased adherence (see chapter 12). When TB patients in Tajikistan were given food conditional on their adherence to treatment, for example, the treatment success rate was 50 percent higher than without the incentive (Mohr and others 2005). In three Russian oblasts, providing a combination of food, travel subsidies, clothing, and hygienic kits if patients did not interrupt treatment resulted in a drop in default rates from a range of 15–20 percent to a range of 2–6 percent (see chapter 12). In the United States, 84 percent of homeless people with a positive tuberculin skin test followed up with medical care when they were given $5 to do so, but only 53 percent did so without the incentive. Regular monetary payments during treatment with directly observed therapy have been shown to increase the rate of completing treatment (Pilote and others 1996; see chapter 8).

Similarly, provider incentives tied to measures such as number of patients cured had a positive influence, although the majority of identified programs that incorporate performance incentives focus either solely on patient behavior or on a combination of both patient and provider behavior (see chapter 12). The Bangladesh Rural Advancement Committee implemented a scheme from 1984 until 2003 that motivated both patients and the community health workers supporting patient care. Patients deposited an initial sum when beginning tuberculosis treatment with the agreement that one part would be returned to the patient at the end and the other would be given to the community health worker (Islam and others 2002). This scheme was ended in 2004 as a condition of receiving funding from the Global Fund to Fight AIDS, Tuberculosis, and Malaria.

Chronic Conditions

About half of the global burden of disease is attributable to chronic conditions and exceeds the burden of communicable diseases in all countries except the poorest.

Addressing chronic conditions such as diabetes, asthma, cessation of smoking and other addictions, obesity, and HIV/AIDS requires significant behavior modification strategies. The evidence about the effects of performance incentives in addressing these conditions comes primarily from developed-country contexts, but hints at the potential (as well as the challenges) in developing-country settings, where control of chronic conditions is particularly important because paying for expensive treatment or losing the household's sole income provider is often an economic catastrophe.

As with TB, performance incentives can improve adherence to AIDS treatment regimens. In the United States, small monetary incentives led to an 18 percent increase in adherence to antiretroviral medication in the short term (see chapter 7). These improvements were not sustained after payments stopped, however.

Independent Health, a managed care plan in upstate New York, used supply-side incentives in a pilot project as part of a strategy to improve the quality of care for diabetes patients. Diabetes was targeted because diabetics were not receiving needed preventive treatment, credible measurement indicators exist, and quality care is critical to medical outcomes. Physicians received bonuses based on a composite quality score of output measures (completion of certain tests) and outcome measures (hemoglobin and blood pressure levels) that conformed to evidence-based recommendations. A package of interventions, such as training and better payer-provider communication, accompanied the bonuses. By the end of the evaluation period, the average composite score for physicians in the project had increased to 48 percent versus 8 percent among their counterparts (Beaulieu and Horrigan 2005). Although the experience is small and the study design is imperfect, the potential for physician incentives to influence quality of care for chronic conditions is clear.

The United Kingdom has used performance incentives to focus attention on gaps in quality. In 2004 the U.K. National Health Service launched the General Medical Services Contract: Quality and Outcomes Framework, which gives family practitioners the opportunity to earn up to a 25–30 percent increase in income if various indicators are met. Evaluations show a positive impact on discrete health outcomes but caution that outcomes might also be attributable to other, simultaneous interventions (Doran and Fullwood 2007).

Demand-side incentives have been introduced to reduce rates of highly addictive behaviors such as alcohol, tobacco, or cocaine use. In general, cash works better than food or other in-kind incentives, and more money works better than less (see chapter 7 for an in-depth discussion). Behavioral changes, however, are not sustained when the payments cease. Despite some indications of success in a systematic review of the literature, incentives do not appear to enhance long-term cessation rates (Hey and Perera 2005). One randomized control trial that examined the impact of performance incentives on asthma-related behavior demonstrated that free medication and transportation assistance significantly increased the likelihood of follow-up, but once again the time-limited intervention did not affect long-term outcomes (Baren and others 2006).

The ability to sustain outcomes is also an important critical consideration. Interventions to reduce obesity are a good example. Studies on the impact of financial incentives on improved weight loss have demonstrated mixed results in the short term, but none has assessed long-term or sustained impacts (Goodman and Anise 2006).

Health System

In addition to promoting health and preventing and curing disease, health sector leaders, policymakers, and the donor agencies that provide support to developing countries often hope to achieve the broader health system goals of increasing use, enhancing quality, and improving efficiency, either within the public sector or by working through contracts or in other ways with NGO and other private providers. To help to reach these goals, performance incentives can be considered on their own or as a powerful complement to other system-strengthening interventions.

In contrast to efforts designed by policymakers and system planners to strengthen health services with brick-and-mortar inputs, training, and information systems, performance incentives catalyze the many individuals and service providers and depend on the ingenuity and resourcefulness of those on the front line. New incentives can stimulate a bottom-up response that results in stronger health systems. In countries with weak regulatory capacity, questionable governance, and spotty records of success with top-down solutions, performance incentives may be especially important to consider.

Increase Use

Increasing the use of preventive and primary care interventions is one of the central health policy challenges in most countries, and performance incentives can be a valuable tool. Because it is typically the poor who use services the least, relative to their needs, the challenge is to design incentives that stimulate either poor households to seek services or providers to make special efforts to attract those least likely to seek care. One approach is to use geographic targeting, which introduces incentives to reward services provided to all people in low-income communities for the diseases that most afflict them. If the incentives improve health outcomes and services, it is reasoned, the poor benefit. A more direct approach is to orient either supply- or demand-side incentives to explicitly reward increases in use by low-income individuals. Performance incentives can also be used to attract health workers to serve the poor and to work in neglected regions.[2]

Demand-side performance incentive schemes are often designed to increase the poor's use of health services by providing rewards that depend on health-related actions that poor households take. For example, CCT programs implemented throughout Latin America have sought to improve equity by providing income transfers to poor households if families keep children in school and take them for preventive health visits. The conditions that tie the transfer to the actions provide an extra incentive to use priority health services. In addition, increased income from the transfers effectively reduces out-of-pocket expenditures and opportunity costs associated with seeking social services. An open question is the extent to which the benefits of a CCT program could be obtained with unconditioned transfers, which would have lower administrative costs (for more on conditional versus unconditional cash transfers, see chapters 5 and 10).

Mexico's CCT program had significant positive impacts on health (see chapter 6). The program increased the use of public clinics by 53 percent overall, decreased the incidence of ill health of children under five years old by 12 percent compared with children not in the program, and improved the nutritional status in 70 percent of participating households. One study found that 80 percent of benefits accrued to families among the poorest 40 percent of the population (DFID 2005).

Nicaragua's performance-based program also used performance-based incentives that were targeted toward poor families (see chapter 11). Using both supply- and demand-side incentives that include paying providers to reach coverage targets, on the one hand, and giving cash transfers to poor households, on the other, Nicaragua's program resulted in an 18 percent increase in immunization levels among twelve- to twenty-three-month-old children, with a disproportionately positive effect on poor households.

---

2. Most conditional cash transfer programs adopt the first approach, using geographic targeting to identify communities in which to intervene. However, the key is application of the performance-based element described in the third approach.

A contracting intervention in Cambodia with some performance-based components is one example of a supply-side intervention that achieved significant pro-poor gains in health (Schwartz and Bhushan 2005). Initiated in 1999 with support from the Asian Development Bank, the management of government-provided primary health care services in Cambodia was contracted to NGOs, which were assigned to the program at random to permit systematic evaluation of impact. One NGO used performance incentives at the staff level to improve motivation and reduce absenteeism among health workers. The contracts with NGOs included a goal of targeting maternal and child health services to the poorest half of the population in each district (Schwartz and Bhushan 2005). The contracting program achieved significant improvements in receipt of vitamin A and uptake of antenatal care and demonstrated the ability to target the poorer half of the population (Bhushan and others 2005).

The gains do not happen without careful design, however. Performance incentives may risk exacerbating geographic disparities in health if not implemented carefully. If the opportunity to earn performance bonuses is greater in areas with higher-income populations, health workers will tend to migrate to affluent regions. In Rwanda, this problem was avoided by giving remote facilities an isolation bonus to mitigate the perverse incentive for health workers to migrate to facilities more likely to receive performance rewards (see chapter 10). Studies by Pieter Serneels and his colleagues show that additional payments can motivate health workers to practice in less desirable, but more vulnerable, areas (see, for example, Serneels and others 2005).

Improve Quality

Performance incentives hold promise for improving both the technical quality and responsiveness of health services. For population-level interventions (such as immunizations) or routine cancer screenings (such as pap smears to detect cervical cancer), quality can be measured by counting how many of these services are provided to the right people. The strategies to do this are the same as those described for increasing the use of services by particular target groups. For more complex interventions (such as antenatal care or appropriate prescription of antibiotics), measures of quality must reflect subtler details, such as whether the diagnosis and treatment are appropriate and clinical guidelines are followed.

Experience using performance incentives to stimulate quality improvements is limited, but some hints of success are emerging. In Rwanda, for example, as in the other known developing-country cases, supply-side performance incentives were first introduced to increase the use of health services. Beginning in 2005, however, the goal of improving quality of care was added in some regions and is now being adopted as a national strategy. Each month, district health teams evaluate the quality of services delivered by health centers using a standardized tool that results in a score. If a facility receives a quality score of 65 percent, for example, it will receive 65 percent of its maximum potential performance payments for that month. This approach was designed to ensure that health facilities focus on increasing both the number and the quality of services provided. Evidence suggests that this strategy is working. An evaluation of early results showed that provinces with incentives to improve quality averaged a composite quality score of 73 percent, while provinces without the incentive averaged only 47 percent (see chapter 10).

In Haiti, responsiveness was measured as an indicator of quality in the first-year pilot of a supply-side pay-for-performance scheme (see chapter 9). A portion of the NGO bonus payment was determined by whether a 50 percent reduction in waiting time for child visits was achieved. However, because the lab services offered by one of the NGOs increased wait times necessarily, program implementers determined that the responsiveness indicator was not measuring quality as intended and dropped it from the payment scheme in subsequent years.

In Mexico, the CCT program was recently evaluated to determine whether improvements in the quality of prenatal care led to positive child health outcomes. Quality of prenatal care was measured using an index of process measures completed by the clinician during prenatal care visits and reported by the mother. The study found that the 101.7 gram increase in birth weight associated with the CCT program was attributable, in part, to improved health care quality. Quality improvements were determined to be responsible for increases in birth weight from 82.8 to 93.6 grams, or a 3.0 to 3.1 percentage point reduction in low birth weight (Barber and Gertler 2007).

Quality of health services is reflected in the proper diagnosis of TB and adherence to treatment through to cure. A review of the evidence of the impact of performance incentives on the detection and treatment of tuberculosis (see chapter 12) found that incentives appear to have beneficial impacts on detection of cases and completion of treatment. In two Russian oblasts, for example, providing patients with material incentives increased adherence to treatment from a range of 80–85 percent to a range of 94–98 percent of the time.

Literature from the United States and United Kingdom frequently cites improving quality of care as one objective of performance payment interventions, whereas improving use is more often the primary objective of performance incentive schemes in developing-country settings. On closer look, however, measures of quality in developed-country settings are broadly defined and often encompass increasing the quantity or use of a particular service considered part of a package of quality care. Rosenthal and Frank (2006), for example, discuss seven incentive schemes that tie rewards to all of the following measures of quality: childhood immunizations and cancer screenings, chronic-care measures, patient satisfaction, investments made in technology and infrastructure, and use of recommended preventive care. A review by the University of Minnesota's Evidence-Based Practice Center examined nine cases of provider incentives to improve quality of preventive care in the United States and assessed quality as the number of patient charts in compliance with a target outcome such as appropriate cancer screenings, weight loss, or immunizations (Minnesota Evidence-Based Practice Center 2004). These reviews report mixed impact of performance-based payment on quality, but because of the broad and variable approaches to measurement, it is difficult to draw lessons about the impact of such incentives on quality that would be useful for developing-country settings.

Increase Efficiency

Performance incentives can motivate individual health workers to provide more services through increased effort with the same level of resources. At the facility level, incentives have catalyzed efficiency gains in how staff are deployed and motivated and have led to innovations in service delivery (chapters 8, 9, and 10). In these cases, providers have implemented novel practices to meet performance targets set by the payer. Hospital reform in São Paulo, Brazil, is a striking example (see box 3-4).

Increases in the number of services provided under a relatively fixed budget are part of what drives improvements in efficiency in most developing-country cases. In the public and NGO sector, where many costs, including salaries of health workers, are often fixed over a period and are unrelated to the volume of services provided, both demand- and supply-side initiatives that increase the number of services provided result in lower costs per service.

Performance incentives offer a targeted way to increase motivation and stimulate innovation. In the Haitian pay-for-performance scheme, for example, the potential to earn rewards motivated individual health workers and inspired efficiency-enhancing organizational change (see chapter 9). NGOs were provided untied budgets and the flexibility to allocate funds in ways the management believed would be most effective. They also had the opportunity to earn

Box 3-4. *Brazil: Performance Incentives for Hospitals*

In the late 1990s, Brazil introduced a set of new public management principles that both gave public agencies greater autonomy and accountability and stimulated results-based financing. Catalyzed by this reform, São Paulo State was the first to establish legally independent hospitals—or health social organizations—financed by linking part of payment to performance targets set by the state. These were set up in sixteen new 200-bed general hospitals, where private nonprofit organizations were contracted to operate facilities financed and monitored by the state. Facilities received a global budget with 10 percent retained until it could be verified that quarterly performance targets had been reached. Health social organizations had full autonomy to make most managerial and purchasing decisions (besides capital investments), including contracting suppliers. While the hospitals were not permitted to charge fees for services, sell services to private patients and insurance plans, or seek outside investors, they could participate in pooled procurement and could outsource clinical diagnostic and hotel services while retaining and investing any savings in capital markets. All health social organizations are in low-income neighborhoods located in urban municipalities on the periphery of the city of São Paulo.

Incentives and Autonomy Equal Increased Quality and Efficiency

A study compared twelve health social organizations to twelve direct administration hospitals of similar complexity and compared performance data for 2003 and 2004. None of the hospitals was a teaching facility, and there was no significant difference between the two groups in the average number of beds, total spending, spending per bed, and number of professionals per bed. The hospitals were also similar in terms of complexity.

In terms of indicators of quality, general and surgical mortality rates were lower in the health social organizations, but the difference was only marginally significant. Pediatric mortality was slightly higher in the health social organizations (2.8 versus 2.6), but the difference was not significant. Health social organizations demonstrated significantly better performance on almost all indicators of efficiency. They use about one-third fewer physicians and one-third more nurses than direct administration facilities. The substitution of nurses for physicians is consistent with international best practice and probably contributes to the lower expenditures, described below. They are significantly more productive in terms of general, surgical, and clinical discharges per bed. Given that average total expenditures are comparable for both groups of facilities, the higher productivity drives lower unit costs. They also spend less per bed-day and per discharge.

What Drives the Strong Performance of Health Social Organizations?

Several reasons have been suggested for why health social organizations outperform direct administration hospitals. First, the newness of the facilities may contribute. Second, they are monitored by state authorities and receive frequent visits from local government authorities from elsewhere in Brazil. This "spotlight effect" may provide a strong incentive for sustained performance. Third, most directors of health social organizations have been in the job since their facilities opened (some have existed for nearly ten years). This is not the case for direct administration facilities, which suffer from high rotation of ranking managerial staff.

(continued)

Box 3-4. *Brazil: Performance Incentives for Hospitals (continued)*

While the previous reasons may explain part of the better performance of health social organizations, it is likely that features of the model also contribute. Key elements include strong decisionmaking autonomy, accountability through a management contract, and performance-based financing.

Findings from an additional study (Costa and Ribeiro 2005) that conducted focus groups, interviews, and surveys with managers indicate that accountability contributes to performance. Managerial authority to recruit, select, and dismiss personnel was an important contributor to success. Findings suggest that an accountability arrangement is at work here that provides incentives to improve quality and efficiency and incorporates five key elements: autonomy, flexible human resource management, strategic purchasing, contract enforcement, and a robust information environment.

Source: La Forgia and Couttolenc (2008).

additional funds linked to the achievement of health targets. The flexibility of funds, in contrast to line-item budgets used earlier, allowed NGOs to concentrate funds on activities that worked and to move funds away from less-effective inputs or practices. Part of their strategy was to share a portion of the NGO-level performance payments with health workers in the form of individual bonus payments.

The same phenomenon occurred in Rwanda, where facility-level performance payments have been distributed partly to staff (see chapter 10). The supply-side incentives in Rwanda stimulated facilities to create their own versions of incentive programs, operating on the demand side. These innovations include paying traditional birth attendants to refer pregnant women for prenatal care and safe deliveries and offering "mommy kits" (a blanket and diapers) to pregnant women as an incentive to deliver in the health center.

Anecdotal experience from some facilities in Afghanistan highlights the importance of motivating health workers in facility-level incentive schemes to achieve performance goals. When bonus payments to health facilities stayed in management's hands and did not trickle down to health workers, the personal motivation of health workers improved very little (see chapter 8). This finding is echoed by a Costa Rican reform, in which hospitals were unable to distribute financial incentives to individuals because of union resistance. As a result, performance rewards retained by management inspired no change in motivation among staff (García-Prado and Chawla 2006).

Demand-side financing also can improve efficiency (Pearson 2001; Sandiford and others 2004). A voucher program for reproductive health services in Kenya, begun in 2006, incorporated performance incentives to encourage providers. In the program, effective demand was increased by using vouchers for a package of prenatal, postnatal, and delivery services to lower out-of-pocket payments. Responsiveness and efficiency were stimulated by allowing women to use vouchers at any of the competing service providers. Participating clinics and hospitals assumed financial risk because they were not paid until the woman had completed four prenatal care visits. Early findings suggest that the competitive pressures among providers result in more attention being paid to marketing and service quality (Bellows, Walsh, and Muga 2007).

Conclusions

The evidence speaks loudly to the possibilities for performance incentives to improve health behaviors and health systems in developing countries. Both supply- and demand-side incentives have been successfully applied to meet the full range of health system goals and to address varied diseases and health conditions. Available evidence suggests that both supply- and demand-side options should be considered during program design, and a mix of approaches might be most effective at changing behavior.

Performance incentives can work in a variety of health systems and contexts. In countries with stable governments that assume some leadership in the health sector, such as Nicaragua (see chapter 11) and Romania (see chapter 12), performance incentive schemes demonstrated improved outcomes for child health and tuberculosis. And in Haiti and in postconflict Afghanistan and Rwanda, where existing state infrastructure was weak and public delivery of health services was failing, performance incentives also succeeded. In these cases, the lack of government intervention may have opened the door to innovations in service delivery by NGOs.

In each of these instances, the public and private sectors had different roles in the provision of health services and the implementation of performance incentives. In Rwanda, performance-based financing was adopted as a national policy, enabling the government to make performance payments to both public and private health facilities after donor-sponsored pilots demonstrated success. In Afghanistan, external funders entered into performance-based contracts with local NGOs and supported development of the capacity of the national Ministry of Health to oversee them. In Haiti, only NGOs were initially contracted using a pay-for-performance model, although Ministry of Health employees are often part of the staff; in 2006 the Haitian government began to adopt the use of performance incentives within public sector facilities.

This chapter has discussed three high-level policy priorities: improving use, quality, and efficiency. Other public health challenges, however, such as fighting drug resistance and stigma, may be opportunities for effective performance incentives. Finding ways to ensure completion of treatment or adherence to drug regimens is critical with infectious diseases, such as HIV and TB, for which the failure to adhere to a regimen can lead to both increased transmission and the development of drug-resistant strains. Performance incentives have demonstrated success at improving adherence to treatment in several cases. With many diseases, significant stigma is associated with a diagnosis. For sexually transmitted diseases, and particularly for HIV/AIDS, cultural stigma inhibits many individuals from getting tested, which means that they do not receive appropriate treatment or counseling to encourage reducing the risk of transmission. Performance incentives are a strategy to mitigate stigma because they enable an individual accessing a diagnostic test to justify taking the test on the grounds of receiving an award rather than on suspicion of actually having the disease.

A common theme among many of the studies cited is that performance incentives are often instituted along with a package of other interventions. Improvements in outcomes are then difficult to attribute only, or even primarily, to the incentive. Further studies designed to isolate the individual effects of performance incentives or, as in Nicaragua, the independent effects of the supply- and demand-side incentives would improve the design of future programs.

Whether a health minister or donor is aiming to improve a country's health system or combat a certain disease, performance incentives can help. Across the experiences presented, we see a few common themes: performance incentives have shown promise in all kinds of places. Both private and public entities have implemented performance incentives successfully. You get what you pay for. And it is easier to pay for what you can easily measure.

Appendix 3-1. *Performance Incentives and Other System Solutions to Solving Health Systems Problems*

Problem and level	Performance incentives	Other solutions
Household or community level		
Financial and physical barriers: households cannot afford to obtain quality care or health care services are hard to reach	*Direct payment for use:* provide incentives to access care by reducing direct costs (may make costs negative) *Transportation subsidies:* reduce direct cost of obtaining care *Food support:* free up income that would have been used to buy food and reduce opportunity costs of seeking care, especially for treatment of chronic conditions *Financial rewards to providers for results (or penalties for poor performance):* motivate outreach, encourage more convenient clinic hours, and stimulate solutions to reduce financial barriers faced by households	*Eliminate or reduce fees:* implement functioning systems to provide fee waivers to poorest and enforce elimination of informal fees *Implement universal coverage:* offer a comprehensive package of services *Build facilities:* enable facilities to function close to where people live; reduce financial barriers by reducing transportation and opportunity costs of seeking care *Regulate quality of low-cost substitutes:* eliminate counterfeit drugs and nonaccredited health care providers through enforcement of regulations
Information and social norms: lack of information and social norms inhibit seeking recommended preventive and curative care	*CCT programs:* often condition payment on attendance at health education sessions; payment conditional on actions can counteract social norms that may drive households to invest less in females; by conditioning payment on receipt of specified services, may alter household decisions to choose low-cost and low-quality substitutes (for example, traditional healers) *Financial rewards to providers for results (or penalties for poor performance):* stimulate improved communication and health education that may enhance care seeking by increasing understanding and reducing social obstacles	*Communicate information on behavioral change:* provide information to encourage healthy behavior *Mandate consumer education:* require health care providers to provide more education about healthy behavior *Have community volunteers provide information:* use community volunteers to convey information close to home about the value of health behavior

(continued)

Appendix 3-1. *Performance Incentives and Other System Solutions to Solving Health Systems Problems (continued)*

Problem and level	Performance incentives	Other solutions
	Regulations that require health screening or evidence of good health as a condition of participation in other valued programs: stimulate changed behaviors, such as regulations that require full immunization as a condition of enrolling in school	
Service provision level Staffing challenges: inadequate supply, maldistribution, poor motivation, and poor quality of care delivered by health workers	*Financial rewards to providers for results (or penalties for poor performance):* can motivate effort and result in innovative changes to the way services are delivered through strategies that may include improved outreach to underserved areas, altered mix of health care workers, and performance awards. Incentives can be structured so it is in providers' interest to adhere to quality standards *National to local transfers based on results:* stimulate solutions similar to the previous item *Demand-side incentives linked to use:* stimulate providers to be more responsive and accountable to households	*Offer training and continuing education:* upgrade skills of existing health workers and train new ones *Alter the skill mix of health worker teams:* maximize effectiveness with the given supply of human resources *Improve health infrastructure and ensure the availability of supplies and medicines:* improve motivation if needed inputs are in place *Pay higher salaries:* improve motivation *Improve management and management support systems:* create, for example, clear career paths, management information systems, stronger supervision, and human resource development systems *Develop quality assurance standards:* develop, mandate, and monitor standards of quality

Appendix 3-1. *Performance Incentives and Other System Solutions to Solving Health Systems Problems (continued)*

Problem and level	Performance incentives	Other solutions
Management challenges: weak technical guidance, program management, and supervision	*Financial rewards to health service–providing institutions for results (or penalties for poor performance):* strengthen management by causing service-providing institutions to examine the range of constraints they face to achieving results and the systems, capabilities, and strategies they need to introduce to achieve them *Demand-side incentives:* stimulate households to hold service-providing institutions accountable for results and, in the process, catalyze a process of strengthening management	*Offer training and continuing education:* offer training in planning, supervision, and management *Set accreditation and quality standards:* institute and enforce standards of accreditation and quality *Improve management systems:* design and implement health management information systems, financial management, human resources management, and drug management *Create provider report cards:* introduce cards to report on provider performance to the population
Drugs and supplies: unavailable drugs and supplies; variable quality	*Drug procurement, storage, and distribution:* contract out the procurement, storage, and distribution of drugs and reward the contracted entity (or entities) based on results *Performance-based incentives in inventory management and distribution:* increase responsiveness by improving management from central to regional to facility levels	*Improve management procedures and systems to strengthen procurement, storage, and distribution of drugs:* reduce stock outs and waste *Improve quality control:* improve the testing of drug quality
Health sector level Resource allocation: inequitable and inefficient distribution of resources for health	*National to local transfers to target services to the poor:* create innovative solutions to increase access and use among the poor and improve equity	*Reform resource allocation mechanisms:* improve equity, target scarce resources to cover the poor, and improve quality

(continued)

Appendix 3-1. *Performance Incentives and Other System Solutions to Solving Health Systems Problems (continued)*

Problem and level	Performance incentives	Other solutions
	National to local transfers on results: improve efficiency by stimulating local solutions *Payments to providers to provide services to the poor:* improve access and equity as part of a social insurance program, a contracting process with the private sector, a system to reward public sector providers, or a combination	*Improve national financial planning:* provide information such as national health accounts and other resource tracking, allocation, and budget allocation
Planning and management: weak and overly centralized systems for planning and management	*National to local transfers based on results:* use transfers based on results to improve planning and management at local levels	*Strengthen management capacities at the central and regional levels:* implement strategies such as training and continuous education *Adopt a national strategy to decentralize planning and management:* transfer management and planning responsibilities to subnational levels of government

Source: Authors.

References

Agüero, Jorge M., Michael R. Carter, and Ingrid Woolard. 2006. "The Impact of Unconditional Cash Transfers on Nutrition: The South African Child Support Grant." Working Paper. Madison: University of Wisconsin. (www.aae.wisc.edu/carter/papers.html [October 2008].)

Baker, Laurence C., David Hopkins, Richard Dixon, Jeffrey Rideout, and Jeffrey Geppert. 2004. "Do Health Plans Influence Quality of Care?" *International Journal for Quality in Health Care* 16 (1): 19–30.

Barber, Sarah, and Paul Gertler. 2007. "Empowering Women to Get Higher Quality Health Care: How Mexico's Oportunidades Program Improved Birth Weight." Working Paper. Berkeley: University of California.

Baren, Jim M., Edwin D. Boudreaux, Barry E. Brenner, Rita K. Cydulka, Brian H. Rowe, Sunday Clark, and Carlos A. Camargo. 2006. "Randomized Controlled Trial of Emergency Department Interventions to Improve Primary Care Follow-up for Patients with Acute Asthma." *Chest* 129 (2): 257–65.

Barham, Tania, Logan Brenzel, and John A. Maluccio. 2007. "Beyond 80%: Are There New Ways of Increasing Vaccination Coverage?" HNP Discussion Paper. Washington: World Bank.

Beaulieu, Nancy D., and Dennis R. Horrigan. 2005. "Putting Smart Money to Work for Quality Improvement." *Health Services Research* 40 (51): 1318–34.

Bellows, Ben, Julia Walsh, and Richard Muga. 2007. "Using Vouchers for Paying for Performance and Reaching the Poor: The Kenyan Safe Motherhood Initiative." Draft note, January 30. Washington: Center for Global Development.

Bhushan, Indu, Erik Bloom, Benjamin Loevinsohn, and J. Brad Schwartz. May 2005. "Contracting Health Care Services for the Rural Poor: The Case of Cambodia." In *Development Outreach: Putting Knowledge to Work for Development.* Washington: World Bank Institute.

Chowdhury, Sadia. 2001. "Educating for Health: Using Incentive-Based Salaries to Teach Oral Rehydration Therapy." Private Sector and Infrastructure Network Note 235. Washington: World Bank.

Christianson, John B., David J. Knutson, and Roger S. Mazze. 2006. "Physician Pay-for-Performance: Implementation and Research Issues." *Journal of General Internal Medicine* 21 (S2): S9–S13.

Costa, Nilson do Rosário, and José Mendes Ribeiro. 2005. "Estudo comparativo do desempenho de hospitais em regime de organização social." Consultant report prepared by FIOCRUZ, Escola Nacional de Saúde Pública, Rio de Janeiro, for the World Bank.

DFID (Department for International Development). 2005. "Social Transfers and Chronic Poverty: Emerging Evidence and the Challenge Ahead." DFID Practice Paper. London.

Doran, Tim, and Catherine Fullwood. 2007. "Pay for Performance: Is It the Best Way to Improve Control of Hypertension?" *Current Hypertension Reports* 9 (5): 360–67.

Dudley, R. Adam. 2005. "Pay for Performance Research, How to Learn What Physicians and Policy Makers Need to Know." *American Medical Association* 294 (14): 1821–23.

Dupas, Pascaline. 2005. "The Impact of Conditional In-Kind Subsidies on Preventive Health Behaviors: Evidence from Western Kenya." Working Paper. New York University.

Fairbrother, Gerry, Karla Hanson, Stephen Friedman, and Gary Butts. 1999. "The Impact of Physician Bonuses, Enhanced Fees, and Feedback on Childhood Immunization Coverage Rates." *American Journal of Public Health* 89 (2): 171–75.

Felt-Lisk, Suzanne, Gilbert Gimm, and Stephanie Peterson. 2007. "Making Pay-for-Performance Work in Medicaid." *Health Affairs* 26 (4): 516–27.

García-Prado, Ariadna, and Mukesh Chawla. 2006. "The Impact of Hospital Management Reforms on Absenteeism in Costa Rica." *Health Policy and Planning* 21 (2): 91–100.

Gertler, Paul J. 2004. "Do Conditional Cash Transfers Improve Child Health? Evidence from Progresa's Control Randomized Experiment." *American Economic Review* 94 (2): 336–41.

Gilmore, A. S., Y. Zhao, N. Kang, K. L. Ryskina, A. P. Legoretta, D. A. Taira, and R. S. Chung. 2007. "Patient Outcomes and Evidence-Based Medicine in a Preferred Provider Organization Setting: A Six-Year Evaluation of a Pay-for-Performance Plan." *Health Research and Education Trust* 42 (6, pt. 1): 2140–59.

Goodman, Clifford, and Ayodola Anise. 2006. "What Is Known about the Effectiveness of Economic Instruments to Reduce Consumption of Foods High in Saturated Fats and Other Energy-Dense Foods for Preventing and Treating Obesity?" Copenhagen: World Health Organization Regional Office for Europe. (www.euro.who.int/document/e88909.pdf [October 2008].)

Guggenheim, Ricardo. 2005. "Putting Evidence-Based Medicine to Work: Easier Said Than Done." *Managed Care Magazine* 14 (12): n.p. (www.managedcaremag.com/archives/0512/0512.contents.html [October 2008].)

Hey, K., and R. Perera. 2005. "Competitions and Incentives for Smoking Cessation." *Cochrane Database of Systematic Reviews* 2 (CD004307): DOI: 10.1002/14651858.CD004307.pub3.

Institute of Medicine. 2001. *Crossing the Quality Chasm: A New Health System for the Twenty-first Century.* Washington.

Islam, M. Akramuhl, Susumu Wakai, Nobukatsu Ishikawa, A. M. R. Chowdhury, and J. Patrick Vaughan. 2002. "Cost-Effectiveness of Community Health Workers in Tuberculosis Control in Bangladesh." *Bulletin of the World Health Organization* 80 (6): 445–50.

Khan, Charles N. III, Thomas Ault, Howard Isenstein, Lisa Potetx, and Susan van Gelder. 2006. "Snapshot of Hospital Quality Reporting and Pay-for-Performance under Medicare." *Health Affairs* 25 (1): 148–62.

Kindig, D. A. 2006. "A Pay-for-Population Health Performance System." *Journal of the American Medical Association* 296 (21): 2611–13.

La Forgia, Gerard M., and Bernard F. Couttolenc. 2008. *Hospital Performance in Brazil: The Search for Excellence.* Washington: World Bank.

Lindenauer, Peter K., Denise Remus, Sheila Roman, Michael B. Rothbork, Evan M. Benjamin, Allen Ma, and Dale W. Bratzler. 2007. "Public Reporting and Pay-for-Performance in Hospital Quality Improvement." *New England Journal of Medicine* 356 (5): 486–96.

Lundberg, Mattias, Tonia Marek, and George Pariyo. 2007. "Contracting for Primary Health Care in Uganda." Unpublished manuscript. Washington: World Bank.

McGlynn, Elizabeth A., and others. 2003. "The Quality of Health Care Delivered to Adults in the United States." *New England Journal of Medicine* 348 (26): 2635–45.

Minnesota Evidence-Based Practice Center. 2004. *Effectiveness of Behavioral Interventions to Modify Physical Activity Behaviors in General Populations and Cancer Patients and Survivors.* Structured Abstract. Rockville, Md.: Agency for Healthcare Research and Quality (June). (www.ahrq.gov/clinic/tp/pacantp.htm [December 2008].)

Mohr, Tom, O. Rajobov, Z. Maksumova, and R. Northrop. 2005. "Using Incentives to Improve Tuberculosis Treatment Results: Lesson from Tajikstan." Millwood, Va.: CORE Tuberculosis Case Study and Project HOPE.

Morris, Saul, Pedro Olinto, Rafael Flores, Eduardo Nilson, and Ana Figueiro. 2004. "Conditional Cash Transfers Are Associated with Small Reduction in the Rate of Weight Gain of Preschool Children in Northeast Brazil." *American Journal of Nutrition* 134 (9): 2336–41.

Pearson, Mark. 2001. *Demand-Side Financing for Health Care.* London: DFID Health Systems Resource Centre.

Petersen, Laura A., LeChauncy D. Woodward, Tracy Urech, Christina Daw, and Supicha Sookanan. 2006. "Does Pay for Performance Improve the Quality of Health Care?" *Annals of Internal Medicine* 145 (August): 265–72.

Pilote, L., J. P. Tulsky, A. R. Zolopa, J. A. Hahn, G. F. Schecter, and A. R. Moss. 1996. "Tuberculosis Prophylaxis in the Homeless: A Trial to Improve Adherence to Referral." *Archives of Internal Medicine* 156 (2): 161–65.

Rosenthal, Meredith B., and R. A. Dudley. 2007. "Pay-for-Performance: Will the Latest Payment Trend Improve Care?" *Journal of the American Medical Association* 297 (7): 740–45.

Rosenthal, Meredith B., and Richard G. Frank. 2006. "What Is the Empirical Basis for Paying for Quality in Health Care?" *Medical Care Research and Review* 63 (2): 135–57.

Rosenthal, Meredith B., Richard G. Frank, Li Zhonghe, and M. Epstein. 2005. "Early Experience with Pay for Performance: From Concept to Practice." *Journal of the American Medical Association* 294 (4): 1788–93.

Rosenthal, Meredith B., B. E. Landon, K. Howitt, R. H. Song, and A. M. Epstein. 2007. "Climbing up the Pay-for-Performance Learning Curve: Where Are the Early Adopters Now?" *Health Affairs* 26 (6): 1674–82.

Rosenthal, Meredith B., B. E. Landon, S. L. T. Normand, Richard G. Frank, and A. M. Epstein. 2006. "Pay for Performance in Commercial HMOs." *New England Journal of Medicine* 355 (18): 1895–902.

Sandiford, Peter, Anna Gorter, Z. Rojas, and Micol Salvetto. 2004. *Voucher Schemes in Health: A Toolkit.* Washington: World Bank.

Schwartz, J. Brad, and Indu Bhushan. 2005. "Cambodia: Using Contracting to Reduce Inequity in Primary Health Care Delivery." In *Reaching the Poor with Health Nutrition and Population Services,* edited by Davidson Gwatkin, Adam Wagstaff, and Abdo S. Yazbeck. Washington: World Bank.

Sedlacek, Guilherme, Nadeen Ilahi, and Emily Gustafsson-Wright. 2000. "Targeted Conditional Transfer Programs in Latin America: An Early Survey." Securing Our Future Paper. Washington: World Bank.

Serneels, Pieter, Magnus Lindelow, José García-Montalvo, and Abigail Barr. 2005. "For Public Service or Money: Understanding Geographical Imbalances in the Health Workforce." Global Poverty Research Group Working Paper Series 018. Swindon, U.K.: Economic and Social Research Council.

Shvarts, Shifra, Jefrey Borkan, Mohamad Morad, and Michael Sherf. 2003. "The Government of Israel and the Health Care of the Negev Bedouin under Military Government, 1948–1966." *Medical History* 47 (1): 47–66.

Sobrero, M. E. S., C. L. Damberg, R. Shaw, S. Teleki, S. Lovejoy, A. Decristofaro, J. Dembosky, and C. Schuster. 2006. "Assessment of Pay-for-Performance Options for Medicare Physicians

Services: Final Report." RAND Health Working Paper Series. Washington: U.S. Department of Health and Human Services.

Thornton, Rebecca. 2005. "The Impact of Incentives on Learning HIV Status: Evidence from a Field Experiment." Harvard University.

Town, Robert, Douglas R. Wholey, John Kralewski, and Bryan Dowd. 2004. "Assessing the Influence of Incentives on Physicians and Medical Groups." *Medical Care Research and Review* 61 (3): S80–S118.

Trude, Sally, and Melanie Au. 2006. "Health Plan Pay-for-Performance Strategies." *American Journal of Managed Care* 12 (9): 537–42.

Wenneberg, John E., Elliott S. Fisher, Jonathan S. Skinner, and Kristen K. Bronner. 2007. "Extending the P4P Agenda, Part 2: How Medicare Can Reduce Waste and Improve the Care of the Chronically Ill." *Health Affairs* 26 (6): 1575–85.

Young, Gary J., Mark Meterko, Bert White, Barbara G. Bokhour, Karen M. Sautter, Dan Berlowitz, and James F. Bergess Jr. 2007. "Physician Attitudes toward Pay-for-Quality Programs." *Medical Care Research and Review* 64 (3): 331–33.

4

Making Payment for Performance Work

The question is not whether performance incentives can—under the right circumstances—change behavior and improve service outcomes. It is "What are the right circumstances?" The answers to the questions of "how" determine the ultimate success, failure, and unintended consequences of performance incentive approaches, yet too often new programs are undertaken without a clear look at the challenges of implementing them.

Here we discuss key issues to consider when designing and the steps to implementing a performance incentives program. Among our examples are those that went wrong as well as those that went right, because valuable lessons can be learned from each. While some of the issues may seem complicated, it is not necessary to get all the details right at the outset: refinements can and should be introduced along the way. Fundamentally different from many traditional approaches to improving the delivery of health services, performance incentives are about establishing what the results should be and then letting the key actors—the patients, the providers—figure out how to achieve them. Along the way, learning and fine-tuning are part and parcel of the process.

The first step is a diagnostic: to understand and determine the major problems affecting performance and to identify incentives that have the potential to inspire the changes in behavior and systems needed to generate positive results. The second is to select service providers and beneficiaries, the results to be rewarded, and the mechanisms to monitor performance. Terms of contractual arrangements, including how recipients will be monitored and performance rewarded, need to be clearly specified. Staff and systems to administer performance-based payments need to be organized, and both technical and financial resources need to be dedicated to assessing, learning, and revising the approach.

Any discussion of how to accomplish all this should emphasize the practical. The decision to introduce a program and the details of design and implementation must balance what might be conceptually desirable with what is actually feasible in a given context. For example, although it may be desirable to foster competition among nongovernmental organizations (NGOs) for performance-based contracts and to have the ultimate penalty of terminating a contract as an option, in some settings only one service provider is present and termination is not an option. Because performance incentive programs are about transferring money and information to change behavior, other factors to consider include the ability to transfer money, the features of existing information systems, political and social realities, and restrictions imposed by donors, governments, and NGO management. Each step in the process must be informed by what is feasible, and making incentives work is iterative rather than linear. Each step is affected by and affects decisions in previous and subsequent steps.

Deciding on the core aims is fundamental; clarifying aims can guide design and implementation and help to persuade decisionmakers that the benefits of introducing incentives outweigh the effort, expense, and possible risks.

In the short term, demand-side interventions, such as conditional cash transfers or the provision of food to tuberculosis (TB) patients, may increase the use of services, improve adherence to treatment, and target resources. On the supply side, performance incentives can generate rapid improvements in the quantity and quality of services, particularly when the starting point is low.

Over the long term, benefits are harder to trace but likely to be real. Nutritious food, more schooling, and income gains within poor households receiving cash transfers can contribute to better health and income potential over a lifetime. Stimulating service providers to improve their productivity and service quality can catalyze changes that strengthen institutional capacity over many years. This dynamic is set in motion when providers start to assess critically whether current delivery approaches will be effective at reaching the selective targets—something they are inclined to do if their income depends in part on reaching those targets. In response, service providers identify system weaknesses and experiment with innovative strategies, such as ways to reach marginalized populations. They may strengthen information and other operational systems to support more effective management.

When multiple objectives are at play, setting priorities is all about trade-offs. For example, if increasing both the use of services and access for the poor is a priority, a program may need to sacrifice some increases in use if the hardest to reach are to be served. The challenge in setting priorities comes when several objectives coincide. Decisionmakers then need to determine the value of each objective. Tools that may be helpful include burden-of-disease analysis, cost-effectiveness analysis, equity analysis, and evidence-based medicine. Because each approach concentrates on only a single criterion, decisionmakers, who must take all criteria into account, need to use a combination of art and science to set priorities (Baltussen and Niessen 2006).[1]

The next challenge is to sort out the problems with performance and what is causing them. If they are the result of provider or patient behavior, then performance incentives can affect results. If they are tied to organization and management, incentives can motivate institutions to change the approaches to care management and the systems and structures that support service delivery. If they are not related to behavior or systems, however, performance-based payments will not help. For example, providers will not be able to increase immunization coverage if they have no access to vaccines and no way to influence that supply. Demand-side incentives will contribute to results only if the supply exists or can be influenced by demand.

Moving Forward

There is no need to wait until everything is lined up perfectly before putting performance incentives in place. Because they bring about behavior as well as systemic changes, incentives can be the catalyst that inspires providers and consumers

---

1. For example, cost-effectiveness analysis is not an effective priority-setting approach if higher value is placed on serving the poor than on serving the general population. In addition, the dynamic responses of providers and consumers to new incentives that result in altered costs are not incorporated. For example, if providers exert additional effort in response to performance awards, their productivity increases, resulting in lower unit costs. Costs may also change if service-providing institutions change the way they organize and deliver care by substituting lower-cost health workers for doctors and working more effectively with communities. Measures of effectiveness do not include contributions to development in areas such as reducing the intergenerational transmission of poverty or strengthening the health care system.

to find solutions in the imperfect environment that is the reality of most developing (and developed) countries.

Identify Stumbling Blocks

Behavior-related causes of poor health system performance fall into two broad categories, which overlap to some extent. The first is having too few resources to enable effective actions. The second is having incentives that work against effective actions. An example from TB control may help to illustrate these distinctions.

Dropout from TB treatment is attributable to a number of factors. On the patient side, low-income patients may not be able to afford transportation to obtain medicines (even when the drugs are free) and may be sensitive to the opportunity cost of lost work. If so, performance incentives can compensate for transportation and lost wages. They overcome the financial obstacle and thus enable low-income patients to get care (*enablers* is the term of art in the tuberculosis community). They also encourage continued patient adherence by compensating for both out-of-pocket outlays and lost income. If the problem is that providers are not motivated to follow up on those who fail to complete treatment, a performance award tied to rates of treatment completion may be effective. Often, a combination of interventions may be appropriate.

New incentives are introduced on top of existing ones, and the interaction is what matters. To build incentives that address poor performance, designers must understand what behaviors the existing incentives are rewarding. On the supply side, the issue is often how individual health workers and institutions are paid. A performance award for providers paid a fixed salary has different implications than one for providers paid through out-of-pocket fees. The proportion of funding that a specific payer represents is an indicator of the likely impact that potential performance awards will have. Providers will consider the effort required, the probability of receiving the award if effort is expended, and the opportunity cost. On the demand side, households and patients will also compare the direct and opportunity costs against the benefits of the incentive. If the expected benefits outweigh the costs, providers, household decisionmakers, and patients will likely be motivated. We discuss how to design the structure of awards later.

Engage Stakeholders

Like any major change in financing, organizing, or managing health services, introducing performance incentives affects many: those who receive the rewards, those who do not, those who benefit or do not benefit from the services provided, and those who administer the programs. All are stakeholders who should be engaged to maximize the effectiveness of a scheme and to minimize possible resistance that may interfere with implementation. Examples to consider include health workers and the unions representing them, umbrella NGOs, consumers, public health workers, managers of health organizations, social and private insurers, employers, policymakers, health department staff, political representatives, and international donors.

Consulting with the recipients of incentives can help considerably in determining the best approach. In Russia, for example, speaking with prisoners to learn what would motivate them to complete tuberculosis treatment after their release led to a program that rewarded completion of treatment with help in obtaining identity cards, which are highly valued because they are needed to secure jobs and housing (see chapter 12).

Stakeholders who are beneficiaries can provide valuable feedback about how the approach is working and how providers are performing. In Rwanda, for example, community organizations interviewed randomly selected households to learn what community members thought about service quality and whether fees to health facilities seemed appropriate (see chapter 10). Subsequent provider contracts were renegotiated on the basis of interview feedback.[2]

Conditional cash transfer programs (CCT) in Mexico, Nicaragua, Panama, and El Salvador have used quantitative surveys and interviews to understand obstacles to service use and to design effective transfers. One question, for example, was whether it is possible and culturally acceptable for women to be primary beneficiaries in indigenous communities. Consultations and focus groups complemented quantitative data to help to determine whether supply or demand constraints, or both, inhibit the use of essential health services.[3]

Effective extrinsic incentives enhance what intrinsically drives people. Health care workers, for example, will react positively to receiving financial rewards for what they already value. Well-designed new incentives can counteract ineffective ones precisely because they help to align behavior with what people instinctively value. A performance-based incentive is also more likely to be consistent with people's values if it is considered fair by those who will or might be affected. Consulting with stakeholders helps planners to understand stakeholder motivations, the incentives that might inspire desired actions, and the potential effects of newly introduced incentives.

2. Description from Robert Soeters, January 8, 2007.
3. Communication with Ferdinando Regalía and Amanda Glassman of the Inter-American Development Bank, October 2007.

Consulting with stakeholders also helps to minimize resistance. In contexts with well-organized health workers, for example, failing to consult with provider associations might generate opposition that could block what would otherwise be viewed favorably (see box 4-1). This is especially important in environments with a history of mistrust between the government or dominant payer and program recipients. Public payers may also object to a change in payment from covering costs to rewarding results because of concerns that providers may earn profits. To overcome such an objection, describing the inefficiencies of the current system and the social gains in paying for results, and discussing how the benefits outweigh the perceived losses, might be helpful.

Market conditions matter. In environments with a dominant payer and many competing providers, the potential for outright resistance is minimized, making it possible essentially to impose a different payment system. In this context, however, consulting with stakeholders is still recommended. A prominent example is the 2006 decision of the U.S. Congress to pay based on performance for services covered by Medicare. Most health care providers feel forced either to play by these rules or to risk losing a large portion of their income. Provider groups have formed in an effort to construct evidence-based indicators and the means to measure performance. In environments with only a few or one provider, the provider has more negotiating power and could refuse new payment terms if it believes that the

---

Box 4-1. *Finding Support among Stakeholders in Kenya*

Managers of a faith-based NGO in Kenya—the Protestant Church of East Africa Chogoria—consulted with their nurses association and local community health committees before introducing performance incentives. The proposed approach was to pay performance awards to rural clinic staff if monthly targets for increased preventive and curative care visits were reached. Concern that paying bonuses to nurses in rural clinics might cause hospital nurses employed by the same NGO to go on strike prompted management to consult with the nurses association. To managers' surprise, the association supported the bonuses because it recognized the hardships associated with living in rural locations as well as how important it was to stimulate stronger preventive and curative care within the community. Community health committees were consulted to identify potential obstacles, explain the scheme, and generate buy-in. Communities were also given a small increase in the proportion of fees collected to maintain or renovate the facility once the clinic had generated enough revenue to cover staff salaries and the costs of medicines.

Source: Eichler (2001).

payer would not want to deny access to services. In this context, consulting with stakeholders helps to generate buy-in and contribute to effective design.

Identify Champions

In most cases, performance-based incentive programs need to be driven by leaders inside a national or provincial health system who are committed to the process. Such individuals are best positioned not only to identify likely proponents and mobilize their support but also to recognize and address potential opponents. For example, in some contexts public sector ministries may see cash payments to providers or individuals as budget cuts and thus argue against the programs. Because change can generate resistance, politically savvy champions can in many environments be critical to success.

Set Funding

The funding for incentive payments may come from existing financial flows—for example, when input-based funding of NGOs by donors is changed to performance-based funding—or it may come from new money as a funding increment on top of existing financing flows. For demand-side transfers, the resources may simply be a new way of using existing social protection funding or may constitute new money for social programs. A situation in which new resources are being added is likely to be the least disruptive, but the incentives will have to be large enough to overcome existing incentives that are embedded within current reimbursement arrangements.

Development assistance for health has expanded dramatically since 1990, from $2 billion to close to $12 billion in 2004 (Schieber, Fleisher, and Gottret 2006). Although not without strings, this increase opens up possibilities to experiment with paying for health. On the supply side, donor programs that provide external funding offer flexibility at the outset. Additional funding could also come from reallocation of public spending, taxes, or donors. Examples include loans from development banks, such as the World Bank–financed program in Afghanistan; funds from bilateral donors, such as the U.S. Agency for International Development (USAID) in Haiti; and funds from external donors, such as the Swedish International Development Cooperation Agency in Rwanda, to support pilot activities.

When providers are offered the possibility of earning performance awards, the total resources required will be affected by the supply response. If performance bonuses are designed as a fee for each additional service provided, for example, the performance-incentive program will require funding for both the incentive and the incremental service provision. If performance bonuses are determined by reaching a predetermined target, the maximum financial outlay can be projected more accurately.

Initiating a new program to contract NGOs and pay based on performance will likely involve negotiations about payment. This will occur in situations when NGOs are selected through competitive bidding and when they are chosen by other, noncompetitive methods. The agreed-on payment charts the course of future financial obligations by the financier for several reasons. The primary one is that reimbursement will be based on demonstrating results rather than documenting expenditures on inputs, which means that the agreed-on bid price becomes the fixed component of the reimbursement providers receive. The bid price may also become the basis on which the performance payment is determined. For example, NGOs in Afghanistan competed to win performance-based payment contracts funded by the World Bank. The bid price became the predictable fixed component of payment and the basis for calculating the maximum performance payment, equivalent to up to an additional 10 percent of the bid price. Changing payment terms dramatically in midcourse can become difficult because of the desire to ensure that the population has uninterrupted access to providers found to be strong performers.

Because few programs are fully new, designing and implementing performance-based payment may need to incorporate rigidities that may have been imposed by history. That is, the ideal approach may need to be tempered by what is feasible given existing constraints. It is often the case, for example, that NGOs and other providers have been delivering services in complex environments for many years, operating with rigid cost structures driven by their current staff mix and other service delivery practices. An adjustment period may be required to allow them to adapt to new payment arrangements. In addition, NGOs that are part of international networks may face externally imposed constraints that may require compromises and departures from what is ideal. Understanding realities of the existing environment through consultations with key stakeholders will contribute to crafting a performance-based payment approach that is feasible to implement.

In addition to the funds needed to reward recipients, the ongoing budget required to run a performance incentive program includes the costs of negotiating, managing, and monitoring performance agreements. It is also likely that additional investments will be needed in the early phases of implementation to strengthen information systems, develop procedures, and communicate the changed incentives to recipients in a way they can understand and act on. In addition to likely new costs resulting from new required capabilities, other costs of running an existing reimbursement system will likely be eliminated. For example, with a change from expenditure-based reimbursement to performance-based payment, there would be a reduction in the costs of auditing financial reports and an increase in the costs of monitoring results.

Select Recipients

The recipient of the incentive, whether individual or collective, should be chosen based on the behaviors that need to change. Acknowledging the reality that trade-offs may need to be considered is critical to an effective program. On the supply side, paying a health worker based on results determined by his or her actions is the most direct way to encourage additional or reoriented effort. However, if what is needed involves teams or a change to the system that delivers the services, a collective approach would be more effective. The choice of recipient should take into account the costs of monitoring performance, and managing payment to different levels of recipients should also be considered.

In some settings there may be no choice of provider. Some regions, for example, may have only one operating provider, and the potential for others to serve that population may be limited. In other cases, performance payments will be provided to public sector workers who are civil servants or to public facilities that are a given. In other settings, the potential gains in terms of lower costs that may result from competition may be offset by the losses associated with communities having to obtain care from unfamiliar providers and establish new relationships and systems with the payer. For example, settings with long-standing relationships between payers and providers—such as the mission sector in much of Africa, which goes back almost a century—may be one case where competition to select recipients may offer few advantages. In other settings, a competitive process to select providers may lead not only to the best results but also to lower program costs. In addition, the possibility that a competitor may apply for a contract to serve a region previously served by a monopoly may impose discipline on a provider that may otherwise have little incentive to change. The decision to use a competitive process to select providers in the beginning of a program is discussed at length in the literature on contracts and is not reviewed here.[4]

Changing providers after a performance-based program is off the ground can present a challenge, or at least entail additional costs, because the new provider

---

4. The decision to use a competitive process to select providers in the beginning of a program is discussed at length in the literature on contracts (see, for example, England 2001; Mintz, La Forgia, and Savedoff 2001; Liu and others 2004; Loevinsohn 2006).

needs both to understand performance-based payment and to build the systems to implement it. In addition, consumers grow to trust and rely on specific service providers, making it difficult to change those providers frequently. Such realities mean that once a provider is included in a performance-based scheme, the right strategy may be to help a poor performer improve rather than to switch to a potentially better one.

Some demand-side incentives are targeted to the household. Others focus on the individual. In conditional cash transfer programs, payment usually is made to the mother because evidence indicates that mothers are most likely to consider the welfare of all family members when allocating resources (see chapter 6). The mother is also often responsible for ensuring that the family meets the performance targets on which payment is conditioned. Some TB programs provide food to households when a family member is sick to compensate for lost income or agricultural production (see chapter 12). Motivating this design choice is the belief that the person afflicted with tuberculosis may abandon treatment to contribute to subsistence of the family when he or she feels better but is not fully cured—an issue especially significant for the poor.

Demand-side incentives are targeted to the individual when individual action or behavioral change is central to attaining the health outcome. Examples include stopping smoking (see chapter 7) and adhering to TB medications (see chapters 7 and 12). If the program targets low-income households or individuals, approaches to identifying the poor include geographic targeting and individual means testing (see, for example, Castañeda and Lindert 2006; Coady, Grosh, and Hoddinott 2004; Lindert, Skoufias, and Shapiro 2006).

Determine Indicators

Indicators and targets for improvement are the backbone of any performance-based incentive system and pose special challenges in settings where information systems are weak and recipients have limited understanding of performance-based payment. The principles are that performance indicators should be relevant, understandable, attributable, measurable, and verifiable.

Relevance speaks for itself: indicators should be related as directly as possible to the objectives and priorities determined by the payer. As far as understanding goes, indicators should be both relatively simple and clearly communicated. If recipients do not understand the performance on which they are being evaluated or how payment is linked to measures of performance, they will not be motivated. Demand-side indicators are usually either actions that households must take, such as bringing a child in for a well-child visit, or proof that a behavioral change has occurred, such as biomedical testing that verifies no use of drugs or nicotine. One supply-side indicator that is relatively easy for programs that seek to improve maternal health to understand is the proportion of deliveries that occur with the assistance of a trained attendant. More complex is a composite index of diabetes care that awards achievement scores for a package of critical targets, both output (such as eye screening) and outcome (such as blood sugar levels below a threshold).[5] Although the latter approach is clearly associated with high-quality diabetes care, it may be difficult to implement.

Changes in performance should, of course, be attributable to recipient actions. If an objective is to reduce child mortality, for example, payment in a supply-side incentive approach should not be based on the outcome measure of reduced child mortality because health service providers do not influence many of the factors that affect child survival. Providers do, however, have a direct influence over whether children are vaccinated and whether the quality of curative care for infectious diseases is high—both clearly and directly related to child health. Thus indicators for these can be constructed. For demand-side incentives, income transfers can be conditional on whether children are fully immunized and receive micronutrient supplements on schedule. These indicators are closely correlated to better child health, yet are under the influence of recipients.

Performance indicators must be measurable and verifiable to avoid disputes between the recipient and payer at the end of a contract period. A clear process should be outlined in the agreement or contract. Indicators that reflect services provided to a large number of people will, of course, show more change and improvement than those that reflect benefits to only a few. Once indicators are chosen, baseline measures need to be established so that targets for improvement can be identified. Results for one period become the baseline for those that follow.

In the early stages, keeping the number of indicators small makes the approach understandable and enables recipients to focus on important changes. Limited experience suggests that more than ten indicators are too many for supply-side programs. Demand-side programs should begin with fewer, although here evidence is even more limited.

The risk to using a small number of indicators is that recipients may focus efforts only on what is being measured and rewarded. The NGO project in Haiti (see chapter 9) implemented a refinement to address this concern. To determine the performance payment, one of two packages of indicators (each including four technical indicators and targets) was randomly selected. This increased the

5. Tom Foels, conversation, October 2007.

number of services that might be rewarded from five to eight and reduced the costs of measurement, because only four indicators were audited and verified. At the same time, uncertainty about rewards caused the expected value of achieving a performance target to fall: to achieve a given effect, the reward has to be higher than it would be without this uncertainty.

From a public health perspective, the best indicators are those that measure whether a desired proportion of the target population is reached. When only one provider serves an area, population-based indicators can be used to establish baselines and targets for improvement in terms of the proportion of a population that should receive a given service—for example, the proportion of pregnant women who give birth with the assistance of a trained attendant. Another option is to establish a target quantity of services—for example, the number of assisted deliveries for a given number of pregnant women. Because providers are not paid unless they reach the target, both approaches encourage providers to develop outreach strategies and to adapt their systems to reach the targets. Approaches that pay for each additional service provided, by contrast, do not provide the same incentive.

Service provider targets can be constructed relative to a provider's baseline or to attain a benchmark of excellence applied uniformly to all. If the goal is to stimulate improved performance of all providers—those beginning with a low baseline as well as the better performers—customized targets may be more motivating to all. A potential disadvantage of this approach is that it may not be perceived as fair if better performers fail to earn bonuses and low performers receive bonuses as they improve.

Schemes that aim to reward only top performance establish a threshold measure of excellence and reward only providers that meet or exceed it. The threshold can be established in advance (immunization coverage must be 80 percent, for example) or calculated relative to the performance of all providers in a network at the end of the performance period (such as only providers in the seventy-fifth percentile of performance measures receive rewards). Given such conditions, poor performers may perceive the probability of success as so remote that they may be unwilling to try to improve, and strong performers may not be motivated to improve. The advantage of this approach is that providers are not rewarded for mediocre performance.

Is there a role for management or process indicators that are several steps removed from health results? The programs in both Afghanistan and Haiti (see chapters 8 and 9) link part of payment to achievement of management targets, such as the presence of a financial management system with specific characteristics (Haiti) or facilities with a tuberculosis register (Afghanistan). One argument for this approach is that part of the objective is to strengthen capacity to deliver health services and that incentives linked to building capacity contribute to this goal. An opposing argument holds that the systems needed to provide improved health outcomes should arise out of innovative responses of the providers rather than a mandated plan. The experience in Haiti suggests that management capacity may increase as part of the institutional response to a reward system focused on health outcomes alone.

Potential positive spillover effects merit attention. Programs that reward delivery of specific services to a target population may lead to delivery of additional valued services that are not monitored. For example, when household cash transfers are tied to child growth-monitoring visits, other problems may be detected during routine visits. Kenya is a useful case in point. Its program providing free bed nets to pregnant women who sign up for prenatal care has documented increased HIV testing, which has prevented the transmission of HIV from mother to child (Dupas 2005).

Determining targets for improved performance is an art as well as a skill, perfected as managers gain experience and programs evolve. Again, indicators should be measurable, and associated targets should be attainable within a contract period.

Monitor and Evaluate

Tracking and validating performance are essential. Information is used to verify whether targets are reached, to monitor what is working, to assess whether changes are needed, and to evaluate the impact of the approach on program goals. Improving the quality and availability of information will likely involve investments in systems to monitor at the level of the payer and service provider. Because performance incentives are introduced when the usual input-based approach does not yield the desired outcomes, the costs of upgrading the information system should be compared to the costs of adopting an alternative approach to improving performance, not to continuing with business as usual.

Linking payment to performance may be a mixed blessing with respect to information systems and how information is used. Managers may be motivated to strengthen the system to track progress toward targets and to identify problems early. However, an incentive may lead to falsifying data to earn the reward, which implies that all systems need a process to validate data as well as to provide sanctions for misreporting.

To ensure that information on supply-side performance is valid, programs rely either on independent verification through population-based surveys, facility surveys, extraction from medical records, and assessments from stakeholders' or providers' self-reported statistics combined with random audits and penalties for identified discrepancies. Independent verification has the merit of not being influenced by the provider incentive and is especially useful in the early stages of a program, when independent assessments of impact can contribute to a decision about whether to scale up and institutionalize the approach.

Basing verification on surveys that collect information from a sample has disadvantages, however, especially as part of a large-scale and institutionalized long-term approach. One disadvantage of a statistical approach is that basing performance on samples implies that the true measure of performance lies within a confidence interval range. It may be difficult to determine whether the measured result is statistically significantly different from the baseline. Another negative is that basing performance assessment on independent surveys does not stimulate the development of information systems in provider organizations to support ongoing management decisions. If one of the goals is to strengthen institutional capacity, payment that is based on provider-reported data with random audits provides a stronger incentive to develop and use information systems than an independent verification approach does. Surveys and other independent approaches to verification can also be expensive.

An alternative is to have providers report their performance and then to subject those results to random audits. In Haiti (see chapter 9), after the initial pilot period, service providers self-reported performance, and an independent firm verified what was reported. This verification included choosing cases randomly, verifying reported summary performance data by checking medical records, and consulting with households to verify that reported services were delivered. The approach encouraged service providers to strengthen their information systems and to monitor progress toward performance targets. This enabled NGO management to identify underperforming service delivery sites early in the process and to introduce interventions to enhance their performance. A disadvantage of this approach is that it captures only those services directly provided and reported on and may not fully capture changes in the delivery of services to priority populations.

Community-based organizations can be tapped to monitor performance in some settings. In the Cyangugu region of Rwanda, for example, local organizations were paid a small fee to conduct interviews with a sample of households. The goal was in part to validate whether the services reported were actually received.[6]

6. Robert Soeters, conversation, January 8, 2007.

Monitoring compliance with demand-side incentive programs is complex, particularly in programs that serve large populations. If the payment is conditioned on whether a service was used, tracking use through household reports carries some risks. Among them is falsified information, which is most likely when household income transfers are tied to it. A more cost-effective option is to rely on provider reports complemented with random checks of evidence from the households. Any verification system should be linked to an effective system of sanctions for evidence of false reporting.

In Mexico, for example, where 25 million people benefit from cash transfers, the national office tracks household compliance and determines who receives payment. Information to determine compliance comes from health providers and flows to local and regional Oportunidades offices, which then transmit reports to the national office. A process to dispute what was reported is also in place to ensure that households are not denied payment in error.

Programs aimed at reducing highly addictive behaviors, such as the use of narcotics or tobacco, have used biochemical confirmation to ensure compliance. For example, as discussed in chapter 7, substance abusers may have their urine tested, and smokers their saliva, as frequently as three times a week. A similar approach used in developing countries uses laboratory tests to verify conversion from infectious to noninfectious tuberculosis. Although intensive biochemical verification is not likely to be feasible in most developing countries, self-reports on behavior could be complemented with random checks.

Define Payment Terms

Any system that conditions some payment on performance targets entails financial risk: payment comes only if targets are reached. It is not clear, however, how much risk is enough to motivate a change in behavior and how much is so high that providers stop providing services.

Experience suggests that risk can be relatively small and still have an impact. In Haiti, 10 percent of payments to NGOs were tied to performance targets until 2005, when the figure increased to 12 percent (see chapter 9). In Afghanistan, nonprofit service providers could earn an additional 10 percent of their negotiated budget if they reached performance targets. In both cases, NGOs had alternative sources of funding, however, making it unclear exactly what proportion of the total came from the performance-based payment program (see chapter 8).

Important design questions involve the terms of the incentive: penalty or reward. Health workers and service-providing institutions tend to respond more positively to receiving additional payments than to losing expected payments. Careful stakeholder consultation can help to predict the likely reaction to different funding arrangements. In Haiti, for example, participating NGOs viewed a combination of withholding and then paying a potential additional bonus as both fair and motivating (see chapter 9).

Performance incentives for service providers can be structured to reward improvement relative to providers' baseline or some absolute benchmark of excellence. The objective may be to improve the performance of all providers or to reward only those that perform adequately and eliminate payment to low performers. These decisions depend on the objectives of the program as well as an assessment of what is feasible, which may include a market analysis of whether it is possible to eliminate low-performing providers in regions where there is only one service provider and others are unlikely to fill the gap.

In environments where there are few service providers—rural areas, for example—improving the performance of existing providers will likely bring more benefits. A hybrid arrangement is also feasible. Combining rewards for improvement with an additional reward for an absolute level of performance may prove worthwhile.

In the developing world, some performance-based schemes have begun by paying additional fees for priority services with the expectation that the additional incentive will stimulate more service delivery. Health workers may understand this approach relatively easily, which facilitates the desired behavioral response. Early pilot schemes in Rwanda, for example, paid a fee for each curative care service and for each vaccination (see chapter 10), fees that augmented other sources of funding.

On the demand side, rewards are often linked to some action taken or evidence of a behavior that has changed. The risk is that the payment is made if the action is taken or behavior is changed, but not if conditions are not met. The ultimate risk is that demand-side recipients, either households or individuals, may be eliminated if the terms of performance are not met. CCT programs, for example, specify a maximum number of allowable absences before income transfers are taken away.

Performance incentives may also motivate unanticipated reactions and have unanticipated spillover effects. Some are likely to be positive, and others are likely to be unwelcome. Careful consideration of all unintended consequences, both negative and positive, should be both part of the design process and incorporated into ongoing monitoring and evaluation. For example, a scheme that rewards only 100 percent completion of treatment may have the adverse effect of causing TB service providers to be unwilling to treat traditionally challenging population groups such as the homeless or substance abusers. Conditional cash transfer programs that base the amount of income transfers on family size may result in families having more children.

Specify Contracts and Agreements

In general, contracts and performance agreements are the instruments used to specify results, how they will be measured, and how payment will be linked to them. Contracts should specify responsibilities, reasons for termination, and mechanisms for resolving disputes.

Many features of performance-based contracts or agreements are similar to those that pay for expenditures or inputs and are not discussed here. Recipient responsibilities include providing the services, reporting, and details such as financial requirements. Payer responsibilities include payment, monitoring, and verification. All contracts should include a process for resolving disputes and give the reasons for termination.[7]

Elements specific to performance-based agreements include performance targets and how they will be measured and validated, payment terms that link payment to results, reasons for termination, and specific reporting requirements. In all these elements, clarity counts and will reduce the likelihood of disputes (see appendix 4-1).

Design Administrative Structure

Performance-based incentive programs break down if not enough attention is paid to how they are managed. Compared to more traditional input-based or fee-for-service approaches, performance incentives require more monitoring and data quality assurance but less attention to accounting for spending on inputs.

The large numbers of transactions in a conditional cash transfer program require attention to the administrative structure and processes that enroll households, inform them of the terms of the program, collect information about compliance with conditions, match what is reported with what is expected, determine whether conditions are met, transfer cash to large numbers of people, and ensure that fraud and misreporting are minimized. Good communication about eligibility criteria and conditions is critical, as are information systems to track enrolled beneficiaries, collect information, compare it with what is required, and issue and reconcile payments (see box 4-2).

---

7. For information not specific to performance-based agreements, see Mintz, La Forgia, and Savedoff 2001; England 2001; Liu and others 2004; Loevinsohn 2006. See also the World Bank repository of contracts in developing countries (http://go.worldbank.org/O2DGFLOYY0 [October 2008]).

Box 4-2. *Managing CCT Distribution in Mexico*

In its conditional cash transfer program, the Mexican government must verify whether each of about one-quarter of households in the country (about 25 million people) meets the eligibility criteria, and it must transfer funds if conditions are met. Every two months, payments are generated for the households that meet program requirements. The lag between verifying compliance and paying the transfers is four months: requirements are monitored in the first month, information is consolidated in the next two months, and households are paid in the fourth month.

To distribute payments to a large number of households, many of which are in remote areas, the government contracted the telecommunications company TELECOMM, which had the required administrative infrastructure and was able to establish local payment points. TELECOMM agents travel to communities on a scheduled rotation, distributing the income transfers. To control potential fraud, TELECOMM receives a beneficiary list from the program with unique holograms that must be matched with an identical hologram in the coupon booklet carried by each household. A local program representative is present when the income transfers are made to resolve disputes. As of 2002, payments were made through a state-owned bank and commercial banks to beneficiaries' savings accounts. By 2005, more than 25 percent of all beneficiary households were receiving transfers directly into their savings accounts. As the volume of transactions grew, other banks expressed interest and new ones were contracted to manage household payments.

Source: Discussions with Carola Alvarez and Ferdinando Regalía, Inter-American Development Bank, February 2008.

Administering demand-side programs that provide food and other material goods faces additional challenges. The difficulties of transporting, storing, and distributing food and other goods are considerable. The tuberculosis program in Cambodia, for example, provides food to encourage patients to complete treatment. As the provision of treatment through outpatient facilities increases, the number of distribution points increases and the number of patients at each facility decreases, posing additional stresses onto an already complicated food distribution system (see chapter 12).

In a program that pays on results, one entity can perform all administrative functions. Alternatively, some (even all) functions can be contracted to a third party. If so, the lead entity will need to manage the contract. For example, in Rwanda, the National School of Public Health is contracted to evaluate provider performance, and in Afghanistan, the Johns Hopkins Bloomberg School of Public Health and the Indian Institute of Management are contracted to assess performance.

Consider Donor and Government Restrictions

Pay-for-performance schemes will be feasible only if they fit within a donor or government framework. Most of these tend to reimburse for documented expenditures and may mandate accounting for how funds are used rather than for results. In addition, governments may prohibit bonuses or supplements to civil servants and may base fiscal transfers on budgets derived from input costs (such as salaries, supplies, and utilities). The rules of the game may need to change for performance incentives to work.

World Bank procurement rules to award contracts to NGOs require competitive bidding, and its procedures do not fit perfectly the typical objectives in a developing-country context, which include strengthening organizations as well as "buying" results.[8] The usual approach is to prequalify a short list of suppliers based on quality and then base competition solely on cost. Another approach uses the model usually reserved for consulting services: competition is based on quality and cost, so that the best value can be selected rather than simply the lowest bid. This approach, called quality- and cost-based selection, was implemented in Afghanistan. In that program, a fixed quarterly payment was made based on the agreed-on price in winning bids plus the possibility of earning up to an additional 10 percent if performance targets were reached.

USAID offers two mechanisms for paying NGOs to deliver services: contracts and grants. Contracts procure services. Linking payment to results is therefore straightforward: fixed-price contracts with an additional award fee that applies when performance targets are met, such as in Haiti. Grants are assistance provided to a recipient with the goal of strengthening capacity or encouraging innovation. Only small grants can be structured to pay based on the attainment of benchmarks.

Government regulations and procedures also pose challenges when pay is based on results. As mentioned, paying bonuses or salary supplements to civil servants is often not an option. One workaround is to establish teams that are eligible for bonus payments. The teams determine jointly how to use the bonus funds, part of which can go to team members. Teams can include all workers in a health facility or hospital ward, for example. Recipients may be required to have a specific legal status to be eligible to receive payments linked to results. For example, in Honduras under the CCT program, implementation was delayed considerably because recipient schools and health posts were not registered legal entities.

---

8. These guidelines were current in 2006, but they may change over time, as donor policies and practices are modified.

Existing national budgeting procedures may pose challenges as well. Line item budgets limit flexibility and autonomy, and uncertainty about the proportion of the bonus pool that will eventually be awarded implies that some money may be left on the table. Adding a line item for performance awards that are conditional on verified results opens the door to an underspent budget, a reality that public officials typically do not favor. An additional challenge arises when results are verified in a period other than that in which the funds were budgeted.

To be able to pay for results, donors, governments, and other payers may need to revise current procurement, budget, and payment procedures. Underlying this change will be a shift from accountability for spending on inputs to accountability for results.

Evaluating Impact

Performance-based payment programs evolve and change as lessons are learned about what works and what does not. The only way to learn is through a well-managed monitoring system that includes ongoing evaluation. This system must go beyond collecting useful, timely, and accurate data: it needs to inform evolving program design.

Performance indicators provide a clear view of progress toward results and offer insight into how the program functions. Also included should be priority services not included in the list of awarded indicators with which to assess possible spillover effects, whether negative, neutral, or positive. In terms of evaluating overall impact, however, a system consisting of routine monitoring will fall short unless data collection is designed in such a way as to attribute the changes in performance solely to the program. Chapter 5 addresses the importance of evaluating impact.

Avoiding Mistakes

Much of this book draws lessons from success stories flavored with a bit of common sense to inform programs in other contexts. There are, though, many valuable lessons to be learned from approaches that did not work. We have identified seven mistakes to avoid when designing and implementing a performance incentive program (see box 4-3).

The first is to forge ahead without consulting key stakeholders. The risks of ignoring this lesson are a program that does not motivate the changed behavior and resistance that derails what might otherwise be an effective strategy. One pro-

---

Box 4-3. *Seven Worst Mistakes in Performance Incentives*

—Failing to consult with stakeholders on the design of incentives, to maximize support and minimize resistance,
—Failing to adequately explain rules (or having rules that are too complex),
—Introducing too much or too little financial risk,
—Having a fuzzy definition of performance indicators and targets, too many performance indicators and targets, and unreachable targets for improvement,
—Tying the hands of managers so that they are not able to respond fully to the new incentives,
—Paying too little attention to systems and capacities needed to administer programs, and
—Failing to monitor unintended consequences, evaluate, learn, and revise.

---

gram in Zambia did not work because those to be motivated were not consulted (see box 4-4). The second mistake is a related pitfall: failing to explain adequately the rules of the game to those whose behavior is expected to change.

The third involves financial risk: both too little and too much can fail. Even if the rules had been well understood, it is very likely that the design of the incentive scheme in Zambia would not have changed behavior because the potential rewards were not significant enough to inspire added effort and innovation. The other end

---

Box 4-4. *Using Performance Incentives to Motivate Health Workers in Zambia*

A scheme to provide performance bonuses to teams working at Zambian health centers was introduced as a pilot program in the mid-1990s. The program distributed quarterly performance awards to the best performing and the most improved of twenty-three centers in the Chongwe District, where 10 percent of fee income remains at the facility level. The other centers received no awards and lost their 10 percent share of the user fees collected. This approach generated no change in staff motivation or health impact. The failure was attributed partly to the relatively short period and partly to design problems.

Among these problems were the size of award (less than $1 per worker per month), the tournament-style competition, and poorly communicated rules. A critical stakeholder group—health center staff—had not been consulted in the design process.

Source: Furth (2006).

---

of the spectrum—too much financial risk—is also a mistake. One NGO in Haiti reduced the fixed portion of the salaries of community health agents by half and offered the other half as a performance award, a level that was too high to be motivating.

Fourth, poorly defined and unreachable indicators and targets are not likely to produce the desired results. Again, in Haiti, all NGOs in 2005 were provided the same performance targets regardless of their baseline, demonstrating that those at the bottom did not improve as much as expected given previous experience with customized targets.[9]

Fifth, approaches that try both to reward results and to specify the inputs to be used to achieve them tie the hands of managers and may thwart performance. Allowing recipients the autonomy to respond to these incentives by using inputs in ways they deem most effective is important for effective implementation (Soeters, Habineza, and Peerenboom 2006).

The sixth mistake is to fail to devote ample attention to the capacity and systems needed to implement performance incentive programs. This includes the details of contracting, establishing indicators and targets and measuring them, transferring funds, and monitoring the successes and aspects that need revision. Failure to pay attention to these details, the seventh mistake, will surely derail what may otherwise be a successful approach.

Conclusions

The decision to pay for results comes when payers are not satisfied and part of the problem is attributable to household or provider behavior or action. Design must be informed both by what is feasible as well as by what is most likely on purely technical grounds to achieve results.

Consulting with stakeholders to identify obstacles to good performance, identify solutions, and generate buy-in is a critical element of successful programs. If stakeholders are not consulted, the chosen design may not change behaviors and thus lead to failure.

The steps outlined—from consulting stakeholders to deciding on recipients, payment methods, indicators, targets, and how to verify results—all take considerable effort. However, they may take no more effort than the alternative approach of pre-specifying the inputs and actions required for the delivery of health services, which

---

9. The Haiti case study illustrates many lessons because of six years of experience with changes, innovations, mistakes, and successes (see chapter 9).

are likely best known by those on the front line. Perhaps most important, the design of performance incentives can and should be an iterative process, because participants learn what works well and what does not, which targets are too easy to achieve and which are too hard, which rewards motivate and which fail to catalyze action. Through trial and error, given good communication with the individuals affected by the incentive program, significant improvements can be made over time.

Appendix 4-1. Sample Contract Provisions for Performance-Based Payment

The following provisions are from a subcontract with a health services organization to deliver a basic package of services with payment determined partly by achievement of results.

Article I: Purpose

The purpose of this subcontract is to introduce performance-based contracting through issuance of a fixed-price, award-fee type of contract. This pilot project is being implemented as a transition from the general, input-based, grant type of agreement to an output-based, fixed-price type of subcontract. After issuing an input-based grant in year one of Project Y, the project awarded two progressively results-oriented, cost-reimbursement types of subcontracts to the subcontractor. The final phase of the output-based strategy is to arrive at a fixed-price, performance-based type of subcontract that motivates the subcontractor to increase its impact in the communes of A, B, C, and D in the areas of reproductive health, nutrition, childhood immunization, and child health.

The contractor shall pay the subcontractor an incentive (award fee) in accordance with the award-fee plan, the objective of which is to increase impact through the subcontractor's technical performance, increase its quality of services (user satisfaction), and improve capacity building in an effort to increase sustainability.

Article II: Period of Performance

The period of performance of this subcontract is June 1, 1999, through March 31, 2000.

Article III: Subcontract Type and Amount of Subcontract

This is a fixed-price type of subcontract with award fees. The fixed price is XX U.S. dollars and is payable for satisfactory contract performance, defined as providing the minimum package of services as further described in Article V: Deliverables. The award fee is YY U.S. dollars and will be paid in addition to the fixed price, provided that the subcontractor's performance accords with the award-fee plan in Article VI.

Article IV: Payment Schedule

Each of the first three payments under this subcontract shall represent 20 percent of the fixed price. They are scheduled for June 1, August 1, and October 1, 1999. Each of the next two payments shall represent 15 percent of the fixed price. They are scheduled for December 1, 1999, and February 1, 2000. The final payment shall represent 10 percent of the fixed price and is scheduled for April 1, 2000. The payment schedule applies only to the fixed price of XX U.S. dollars. An award-fee board shall be established to determine the award amount that the subcontractor may earn in whole or in part at the end of the period of performance. The award-fee board shall be composed of at least three members of the contractor's staff. The contractor shall evaluate the subcontractor's technical performance against the performance indicators specified in the award-fee plan in Article VI. The amount of the award fee to be paid to the subcontractor shall be a determination unilaterally made by the award-fee board and is not subject to the disputes clause. Payment of the award fee shall be made after the expiration date of this subcontract and as soon as the results of local impact surveys are received.

Article V: Deliverables

Under the project, the subcontractor shall provide to a population of approximately 160,560 residents in the communes of A, B, C, and D the minimal package of services as described in the strategy document for 1998–2000. The subcontractor agrees to provide the staff necessary to prepare and conduct biannual, joint assessments of service delivery with the contractor. The subcontractor's staff shall participate in discussions with the contractor regarding the results of the assessments, programmatic changes, plans for sustainability of revenue generation, and related management issues during the pilot phase of this performance-based contract.

During this pilot phase, the subcontractor agrees to participate in the performance-based cluster group to review strategies and document the experience. If the volume of services at any time during this period falls below 80 percent of the expected trend (based on historical data), the subcontractor agrees to meet with the contractor to discuss the situation and define corrective measures. If the downward trend continues, the contractor reserves the right to reverse this subcontract to the previous cost-reimbursement type of contract. In any case, the total amount of this subcontract for the period February 1999–March 2000 will be no more than the total approved in January 1999. The subcontractor agrees to participate in the technical assistance activities organized under the project for this pilot phase.

Article VI: Award-Fee Plan

At the end of the contract period (March 31, 2000), the achievement of indicators described in the following list will be assessed. A yes or no decision will be made for each indicator in the list.

The total award fee will be calculated based on the relative weight of indicators for which the subcontractor has met the agreed targets.

Selected Indicators and Targets for Performance-Based Financing

The following list includes the selected indicators, expected results, and their relative weights that form the basis for assessing the performance of the subcontractor under this subcontract. Although estimated levels of those indicators exist, it is considered convenient to validate the actual baseline measurement of each of the indicators during the first month of execution of this contract. The project is directly responsible for financing that validation activity.

1. Percentage of women using oral rehydration solution (ORS) for children with diarrhea. The expected result is a 15 percent increase in use of ORS. Full achievement of the target will earn 10 percent of the total additional award in this contract. The current baseline value for this indicator is estimated at 65 percent in the area being covered.

2. Full vaccination coverage for children twelve to twenty-three months. The expected result is a 10 percent increase in vaccination coverage. Full achievement of the target will earn 20 percent of the total additional award in this contract. The current baseline value for this indicator is estimated at 63 percent in the area being covered.

3. *Coverage of pregnant women with three or more prenatal visits; includes home visits in cases of women missing visits (if the indicated service is provided during the visit).* The expected result is a 20 percent increase. Full achievement of the target will earn 10 percent of the total additional award in this contract. The current baseline value for this indicator is estimated at 45 percent in the area being covered.

4. *Number of institutional service delivery points (ISDPs) that provide four or more modern methods of contraception, and number of outreach points that provide three or more modern methods, at a significant level (5 percent or more of method mix).* The expected result is to have all ISDPs providing four or more methods and 50 percent of outreach points having at least three modern methods. Full achievement of the target will earn 20 percent of the total additional award in this contract. The current baseline values for this indicator are estimated in two of five ISDPs that are already providing expected family planning services; ten of sixty-five outreach points for delivering services are already providing the expected program performance in the area covered.

5. *Level of discontinuation rate for injectable and oral contraceptives.* The expected result is a 25 percent reduction in the level of discontinuation. Full achievement of the target will earn 20 percent of the total additional award in this contract. The current baseline value for this indicator is estimated at 35 percent in the area being covered.

6. *Average duration of waiting time before providing appropriate attention to a child (in hours and minutes from arrival to beginning of attention).* The expected result is a 50 percent reduction. Full achievement of this target will represent 10 percent of the total additional award in this contract. The current baseline value for this indicator is estimated at forty minutes (as an average) in the area covered.

7. *An effective system for supervision.* The expected results are (a) existence and use of a protocol for supervision; (b) development of a supervision calendar at the institutional and community levels, with the results reported quarterly; (c) records documenting supervision visits to 100 percent of staff. Full achievement of this target will earn 10 percent of the total additional award in this contract. The current baseline value for this indicator is a supervision system that is not clearly defined, consistently implemented, or used to manage or improve performance.

At the beginning of the pilot program, Agency Z will measure baseline values in collaboration with the subcontractor to validate the baseline estimates. If the study indicates significant differences between these measurements and the initial baseline estimate, the contractor and the subcontractor agree to immediately revise these targets. Once the contractor and the subcontractor agree on the actual baseline measurement, any change in those indicators must be made by issuance of an amendment under this subcontract.

Article VII: Technical Direction

Performance of the work herein shall be subject to the technical directions of the chief of party or his delegate. As used herein, "technical directions" are directions to the subcontractor that amplify project descriptions, inputs, activities, and objectives; suggest project directions; or otherwise inform and complete the general scope of work. "Technical directions" must be within the terms of this subcontract and shall not change or modify them in any way.

Article VIII: Technical Reports

Monthly statistical reports are to be submitted to the project offices within fifteen days after the end of the month and shall follow the standardized format set forth by the contractor. Three quarterly management reports and one final report shall be submitted within fifteen days of the end of the quarter. The reports shall focus on management decisions made to address cost efficiency, strategies in program sustainability, and an indication of the amount of program income generated and the activities supported by the program income. The quarterly management reports should also illustrate how the overall project budget has been utilized by the sub-contractor to incorporate efficiency in management performance.

Source: Eichler and Aitken (2001).

References

Baltussen, Bob, and Louis Niessen. 2006. "Priority Setting of Health Interventions: The Need for Multi-criteria Decision Analysis." *Cost Effectiveness and Resource Allocation* 4 (14): doi:10.1186/1478-7547-4-14.

Castañeda, Tarsicio, and Kathy Lindert, with Benedicte de la Briere, Luisa Fernandez, Celia Hubert, Osvaldo Larranaga, Monic Orozco, and Roxana Viquez. 2006. "Designing and Implementing Household Targeting Systems: Lessons from Latin America and the United States." Paper presented at the Third International Conference on Conditional Cash Transfers, Istanbul, June.

Coady, David, Margaret Grosh, and John Hoddinott. 2004. *The Targeting of Transfers in Developing Countries: Review of Experience and Lessons.* Washington: World Bank.

Dupas, Pascaline. 2005. "The Impact of Conditional In-Kind Subsidies on Preventive Health Behaviors: Evidence from Western Kenya." Working Paper. New York University.

Eichler, Rena. 2001. "Performance-Based Reimbursement of Rural Primary Health Care Providers: Evidence from Kenya." Presented at the Third International Health Economics Association World Congress, York, U.K., July.

Eichler, Rena, and Riita-Liisa Kohlemainen Aitken. 2001. "Using Performance-Based Payments to Improve Health Programs." *The Manager: Management Sciences for Health* 10 (2): 1–22. (erc.msh.org/TheManager/English/V10_N2_En_Issue.pdf [October 2008].)

England, Roger. 2001. *Contracting and Performance Management in the Health Sector: A Guide for Low- and Middle-Income Countries.* DFID Health Systems Resource Centre. London: DFID.

Furth, Rebecca. 2006. *Zambia Performance-Based Incentives Pilot Study Final Report.* Washington: USAID and the Quality Assurance Project. (www.qaproject.org/news/PDFs/ZambiaPerformancePilotStudyInitiatives.pdf [October 2008].)

Lindert, Kathy, Emmanuel Skoufias, and Joseph Shapiro. 2006. *Redistributing Income to the Poor and the Rich: Public Transfers in Latin America and the Caribbean.* SP Discussion Paper 0605. Washington: World Bank.

Liu, Xingzhu, David R. Hotchkiss, Sujata Bose, Ricardo Bitran, and Ursula Giedion. 2004. *Contracting for Primary Health Services: Evidence on Its Effects and a Framework for Evaluation.* Bethesda, Md.: Partners for Health Reform*Plus,* Abt Associates.

Loevinsohn, Benjamin. 2006. *A Toolkit on Contracting for Health Services in Developing Countries.* Discussion draft. Washington: World Bank.

Mintz, Patricia, Gerard La Forgia, and William D. Savedoff. 2001. *Contracting Health Services: Getting from Here to There.* Washington: World Bank.

Soeters, Robert, Christian Habineza, and Peter Peerenboom. 2006. "Performance-Based Financing and Changing the District Health System: Experience from Rwanda." *Bulletin of the World Health Organization* 84 (11): 884–89.

Schieber, George, Lisa Fleisher, and Pablo Gottret. 2006. "Getting Real on Health Financing." *Finance and Development* 43 (4): 46–50.

5

A Learning Agenda

What elements of performance incentive programs lead to success? What pitfalls can be avoided? When do performance-based programs generate more bang for the buck than other approaches? What tools are needed to help governments and nongovernmental organizations (NGOs) put performance-based financing in place? Moving beyond the monitoring and evaluation that should be a part of any performance-based program (chapter 4), here we propose an agenda for learning that extends beyond any individual country or program. It is about developing knowledge and tools that can be used widely, rigorously measuring and understanding what works across settings, and creating an ongoing way to share and learn among those who are implementing and studying performance-based programs.

Filling the Toolbox

Our look at several real-world cases suggests that three types of new tools would be particularly useful in strengthening future programs.

Standardized Assessments

To date, most performance-based initiatives in the developing world have focused on either overcoming household- or patient-related barriers or changing provider reimbursement to affect the behavior of individual health workers, managers, and the systems to deliver services. Few have tackled both at the same time. The choice—demand, supply, or both—has rarely been driven by an explicit assessment of all barriers; instead, it has usually been based on the starting premise and mandate of the designers. Even more neglected are the actions required by other actors, such as other sectors or community-based initiatives, to support the effective use of essential interventions. A comprehensive assessment of the causes of poor performance would be a sound first step toward designing performance-based programs.

Such an assessment might include the following:

—Methods to measure the extent of problems with use, efficiency, and quality of service,

—Diagnostic questions, analysis, and qualitative methods to assess provider productivity and quality and to understand existing incentives and their effects on behavior,

—Analysis of household survey data to quantify household barriers to effective use of health services,

—Diagnostic questions to clarify objectives and prioritize problems that the incentives would address,

—Analytic tools, such as worksheets, to estimate the costs of implementing a performance-based program, both the near-term costs of switching and the likely recurrent costs,

—Guidelines for mapping the interest groups likely to favor or oppose a performance-based incentive approach, and

—Tools to model the potential impact of incentives, such as a simulation model to ask "what if" under various assumptions.

A related tool with some of these features has been developed, field tested, and refined for tuberculosis control programs (see Weil and others 2004). This could be adapted for other applications.

Performance Indicators

A dynamic handbook on performance indicators would address the challenge of selecting which indicators are appropriate in given circumstances. Such a volume would also bring together the best available evidence about the link between desired health outcomes and particular observable behaviors that might be changed with the introduction of incentives. This is particularly important for provider-side interventions, which often seek not only to increase the use of key services but also to improve the quality of service delivery. Approaches to measuring responsiveness and satisfaction of households would also be included, with sample instruments to measure user satisfaction that could be implemented cost-effectively at the community or service provision level. The starting point would be to develop a set of evidence-based process and output measures related to quality, drawing from evidence-based guidelines and consumer assessment instruments.[1]

The handbook could also provide guidance on methods to measure and validate performance that are feasible in developing-country contexts, including approaches to measuring and validating performance that can be implemented in countries with paper medical records and limited access to technology. Specifications needed to measure and validate results through an independent third party and systems for recipients to self-report coupled with random audits could also be included. Step-by-step guides to monitor and verify results that could be adapted to a specific context would reduce start-up costs.

Contracts and Agreements

A compendium of contracts and performance agreements detailing how payment is linked to performance would provide a useful menu of options. Included could be contracts that specify performance indicators and targets, how performance is measured, and how payment is linked to results. The contracts might also incorporate notes from the designers and implementers that explain why the specific indicators and payment approaches were chosen and the reasons for modifications and lessons learned during implementation.

The handbook and compendium of contracts could be organized as online resources, be updated at relatively low cost, and invite contributions from researchers, practitioners, and others. The online documentation could be supplemented by occasional expert panel reviews of indicators and terms of the contract.

Assessing the Impact

Financiers, governments, and policymakers at every level want to know which approaches to paying for performance have the greatest impact and when paying for performance is more effective than other approaches. They would also like to avoid the failures of other performance incentive programs and replicate the

---

1. Websites include www.who.int/child-adolescent-health/publications/pubIMCI.htm, ih.jhsph. edu/chr/fhacs/imci2.htm [October 2008], and www.ebmny.org/cpg.html [October 2008].

successes. To address those needs, we can examine, closely and rigorously, the effects of relevant alternative approaches, to establish a causal link between programs and outcomes. Analyzing program performance after the fact through routine program monitoring data and quasi-experimental research methods is productive, but subject to biases that are difficult to correct and therefore make it hard to draw reliable conclusions.

To measure the impact of a new program, it is best to observe the same individuals or providers in parallel situations, with and without the program, at the same time. The comparison group can be created any number of ways, including random assignment, statistical matching, and eligibility filtering. Of these, random assignment is most likely to avoid biased results, although obstacles to its use in many settings are significant. Such an approach enables us to account for other factors that may determine success of those in the program, such as whether more capable providers—those most likely to be high performers without additional financial incentives—elect to participate.

In all the cases highlighted in this book, packages of interventions were implemented simultaneously, making it hard to attribute an improvement in performance to any one of them. For example, many supply-side programs include technical assistance, increased funding, strengthened information systems, increased autonomy, and precise definition of expected results accompanied by improved monitoring. Is improved performance coming from the financial incentive, the clear expectations, the better information, or the increased autonomy? Most likely, it is attributable to a combination of factors, and the package as a package is the relevant intervention to examine, not individual elements. More information is needed, though, to disentangle the contributions of interventions that are introduced simultaneously.

The Nicaragua program faced an additional challenge because it included both supply-side and demand-side incentives. Its impact evaluation examined the impact of the package but did not disentangle the contribution of the elements. To establish the relative importance of different interventions, different treatments, such as technical assistance, funding, and technical assistance plus funding, would have to be compared against each other and a comparison group. Choices among possible comparisons to study should be based on real-world options.

Impact evaluation is more than a tool for gauging impacts at the end of a program and providing inputs into a cost-effectiveness analysis. It can also help a program to evolve. For example, in the initial phase of a pay-for-performance program, three contracts with different risk levels can be piloted. Based on the results from an early evaluation, the most effective contract can be scaled up. Several parameters lend themselves to this kind of experimentation, including the relative effects of supply versus demand interventions, the level of rewards offered for performance, and the balance of trade-offs between access and use.

In addition, impact evaluations should collect data to allow for possible unintended perverse or positive effects. Monitoring to determine whether increased attention on rewarded services leads to neglect of other important services is critical. The impact on the distribution of health workers also requires careful assessment because the potential to earn performance awards can either exacerbate or mitigate regional differences, depending on the design. Careful monitoring and evaluation can help to identify positive spillover effects such as an increased use of services, rewarded and not, by a previously underserved population group.

On a local level, impact evaluation can be valuable in maintaining and strengthening political support. In addition, although no findings from one context can be generalized without qualification, the impact evaluation of one program does provide valuable lessons, such as a benefit that is amplified as evidence from a number of similar programs is combined. A good example on the demand side is conditional cash transfers (see chapter 6). For other demand-side interventions, however, as well as for most supply-side interventions, the evidence remains thin.

Evaluations that provide lessons for other contexts ideally would describe the market for services—number of providers, potential for competition—that existed before and the problems and constraints that the incentives were designed to address. A description of the landscape of service provision that includes the number of providers serving a given population would be useful contextual information.

Understanding the incentives that providers faced before performance incentives were introduced may enable insights into the applicability of a given experience to another context. Environments in which providers are paid a salary not linked to performance differ from those in which they are given capitation payments or fees. The new incentives interact with the existing incentives. A program that pays performance awards by holding back or reallocating money from existing budgets may affect behavior differently than a program that funds performance awards by using new funding. The same design, for example, might have desired effects when funded by infusing new money and weak effects when funded by reducing existing budgets. Although the source of funding is not likely to be an element of an impact evaluation in a specific environment, it is an element of design and context that needs to be noted when building a global body of evidence.

When to Consider Programs

Performance incentives are one in a basket of potential approaches to improve health results. How do donors and policymakers choose? Key to this decision is whether and under what circumstances using money to buy results generates a higher return. Evaluations are needed that compare performance incentives to training and other approaches.

Another important question is whether the benefits justify the costs incurred. In addition to immediate-term benefits, such as increased use of services, performance incentives may provide benefits that will be realized only over decades, such as strengthening the capacity of delivery systems and alleviating poverty. Comparisons of alternate interventions need to attempt to capture such multiyear benefits.

Key Questions

Impact evaluations and other research efforts are most useful when they address questions that can inform future design and implementation decisions. Future research might well incorporate and examine the questions that follow, which are in no way intended as comprehensive.

—*Demand-side programs*. The magnitude of financial transfers needed to achieve health goals,[2] whether the costs of conditioning payment justify the benefits, whether communicating the conditions of income transfer without monitoring compliance is enough, how changes in demand affect provider actions, and whether there are unintended consequences and effective strategies to avoid negative effects.

—*Supply-side programs*. The effects and costs of providing incentives to individuals and to teams, the advantages and disadvantages of schemes that pay for each service over those that pay on the basis of population-based targets or a balanced score card, the share of provider income to be at risk and the form pay-

---

2. An impact evaluation is being implemented in Malawi that is examining the effect of none to significant financial payments to people who are HIV negative if they maintain their negative status after one year. People are randomly assigned at the point of their HIV test to payment regimes that vary from no payment to the equivalent of two months' average wage. In addition to providing information about whether performance incentives work, this study will provide more refined information to inform how much payment yields the desired result and whether there are diminishing returns (Rebecca Thornton, discussion, December 2007).

ment should take, the best target-setting strategy (provider baseline, absolute threshold, tournament style, or a combination), the effects of implementing a program by reallocating existing budgets and by using new funding, and how to avoid negative effects and enhance positive effects.

Creating a Network

Some of the most important knowledge needed for successful performance-based incentive programs will be gained by trial and error and be captured by those undertaking the challenge of implementing programs. A serious global learning agenda should include creating a learning network of funders, researchers, and program managers across countries.

A starting point might be an interactive website offering an "ask the expert" series, case studies, and a library of performance incentives. As incentive programs grow and lessons accumulate, the benefits of global networking to share lessons will also grow.

Likely candidates for a network approach include supply-side strategies that provide performance-based payment at the institutional level or higher. A network of payers might also be a helpful way for a range of programs to learn from one another. National programs that implement performance-based payment programs can benefit from cross-country networks to exchange lessons. For example, tuberculosis control programs that have implemented some form of either supply-side or demand-side incentives have met three times at the annual meeting of the International Union Against Tuberculosis and Lung Disease to share lessons and to reach consensus on incentive approaches that increase both case detection and treatment completion. The World Bank has organized international meetings that bring together delegations from across the globe to discuss conditional cash transfer programs. Officials and researchers from Mexico, Chile, Brazil, Argentina, and Colombia meet frequently to exchange lessons about CCT programs, and Mexico frequently hosts delegations from other countries wishing to view the program in action.

Conclusions

The learning agenda set out here is ambitious and important. It calls for new tools to help practitioners to implement performance incentive programs and to link people across the globe in a dynamic and interactive framework that allows them to share and learn from one another. It also calls for a commitment to conduct impact evaluations that will generate the sound body of evidence needed if financiers and program implementers are to understand whether and when there is value in paying for results.

Reference

Weil, Diana, and others. 2004. "Mapping the Motivations of Stakeholders to Enable Improved Tuberculosis Control: Mapping Tool for Use in Workshops." Arlington, Va.: Management Sciences for Health and the Stop TB Partnership.

PART TWO

Case Studies

The chapters that follow provide in-depth looks at a broad range of performance-based approaches and attempt to give a sense of the design and operational issues involved in establishing functional incentive programs. We look at incentives operating on the demand side, such as conditional cash transfers; those that are focused on directly changing provider behavior, such as the programs in Haiti; and programs that combine both supply- and demand-side approaches (such as in the Nicaragua case).

The studies show that well-designed incentives can increase use, quality, and efficiency in a variety of situations:

—In fragile and more stable states, nongovernmental organizations (NGOs) have been contracted and paid based on results. Pay for performance provides a way to establish leadership of a nascent government, while building on existing capacity to deliver services (Afghanistan), and works in settings where the government is not able or willing to take the lead (Haiti).

—In decentralized and centralized contexts, incentives provide a way to establish Ministry of Health leadership and ensure a focus on health results while shifting operational responsibility to lower levels.

—In very poor countries and in the most developed countries, across varying capacity constraints, pay for performance can be both pro-poor and equity enhancing.

The scale of interventions in these cases also varies: some, such as Haiti and Rwanda, start with small pilots, whereas others, such as Afghanistan, are implemented at full scale.

The cases demonstrate that paying for performance is a development strategy about more than buying results today. It can be about strengthening capacity to deliver services by enhancing systems for the long haul—raising health status for the long run, a necessary building block for any country's long-term development.

6

Latin America:
Cash Transfers to Support Better
Household Decisions

Amanda Glassman, Jessica Todd, and Marie Gaarder

Highlights

Conditional cash transfers (CCTs) in Latin America have been effective at increasing the use of preventive health services, increasing knowledge, improving attitudes and practices, enhancing nutritional status, and reducing morbidity, mortality, and fertility.

Rigorous impact evaluations suggest that improved health results can be attributed to demand-side performance incentives.

Better choice of health conditionalities in future CCT programs could strengthen the impact on health.

Poor families in the developing world face significant constraints in accessing essential health care. Distance to health facilities, lost wages associated with illness, care taking and care seeking, facility fees, and other out-of-pocket costs all contribute to limiting the access of poor families to health care, particularly

The authors thank Marcus Goldstein, Rena Eichler, Ruth Levine, and other members of the Center for Global Development's Performance-Based Incentives Working Group for their comments. The research assistance of Lucía de la Sierra is also appreciated.

preventive care. These costs also affect their financial security because out-of-pocket spending can drive them deeper into poverty.

Counteracting these constraints requires a multipronged strategy aimed at both the supply and the demand sides of a health system. Here we focus on a demand-side program known as a conditional cash transfer (CCT). CCT programs are spreading rapidly through the developing world. Since 1997, seven countries in Latin America and the Caribbean have implemented and evaluated CCT programs with health and nutrition components. These include the Bolsa Alimentação/Bolsa Familia in Brazil, Familias en Acción (FA) in Colombia, the Bono de Desarrollo Humano in Ecuador, the Family Allowance Program (PRAF) in Honduras, the Poverty Alleviation through Health and Education (PATH) in Jamaica, Progresa and Oportunidades in Mexico, and the Red de Protección Social (RPS) in Nicaragua. Others are being developed in Argentina, Chile, Costa Rica, El Salvador, Panama, Paraguay, and other countries around the world.

CCTs aim to stimulate demand for health services by transferring cash to poor mothers conditional on their seeking services at clinics and attending health education talks. Because the transfers are conditional, CCT programs also are designed to induce changes in health and nutrition behavior; they are demand-side payments for performance, where performance is healthy behavior.

The central objective is to reduce poverty. A second set of objectives relates to increased food consumption, school attendance, and use of preventive health care among the poor. In the longer term, CCT programs are expected to contribute to increasing human capital and the associated returns in the labor market by reducing malnutrition and improving health and schooling completion rates. Although we focus on the impact of these programs on health and nutrition, the impacts on poverty, inequality, and schooling are also critical to consider when calculating the costs and benefits of CCTs.

A key feature of CCT programs is the rigor with which they have been evaluated. First undertaken in Mexico, an experimental evaluation design showed that significant impacts on social welfare could be attributed to conditional cash transfers to poor families. They have been adopted widely in part because there is solid evidence of their success.

Program Effect Model

Understanding the causal pathways of an intervention is critical to evaluating how it works and what should be modified to improve its effectiveness.

Demand- and Supply-Side Factors

Whether people use health services is determined by a combination of demand-side and supply-side factors.[1] Illness reduces productivity, the time available for production, and individual well-being. To minimize these effects, individuals tend to invest in their health to be healthy or at least to regain their health after an illness.[2] The extent to which the desire to invest results in demand for health care depends on whether an individual identifies illness and is willing and able to seek appropriate care (Ensor and Cooper 2004). Identifying illness may depend on both the type of illness and the individual's knowledge. Willingness to seek care is affected both by knowledge and perceptions (social norms) and by the costs of seeking treatment, household income, quality and availability of substitute products and services, and decisionmaking within the household.

As Eichler (2006) noted, the supply of health care services is determined by a combination of structural inputs (staff time, infrastructure, drugs, supplies, and land, for example) and the processes that transform these inputs into outputs (that is, available technology and the management capability of the provider). Central to this transformation is the behavior of the health care provider. At the individual level, providers have a desire to make money and have leisure time as well as to cure patients. Deficiencies in the quality of care are thus associated with inappropriate incentives for providers, along with inadequate resources, organizational rigidities, and lack of knowledge.

Assumptions

At least nine implicit assumptions underlie the design of CCT programs. The first is that the poor underuse existing health services. The decision to condition payments on having regular checkups at a health clinic is based on this assumption.

Baseline documentation of health and nutrition in countries with CCT programs indicated significant inequalities in the use and fiscal impact of health care by socioeconomic strata. Poor and rural households were much less likely to

---

1. The typical CCT program in Latin America has tended to include little in terms of direct supply-side interventions (Nicaragua is the exception) and has involved intersectoral agreements with ministries of health to provide services to program beneficiaries. In some countries, this commitment is made more explicit by tagging the budget line going to the health sector so that it is earmarked for CCT program beneficiaries.

2. These ideas were presented in an article by Mushkin (1962) and formalized by Grossman (1972).

identify illness and seek care than their better-off counterparts. Out-of-pocket spending on health was a larger proportion of total expenditures among the poor than among the wealthy. In addition, costs associated with seeking care were frequently cited as a reason for not using services. Even in systems with strongly progressive public spending on health, the poor displayed lower use rates.

Little analysis, however, has been conducted to test the proposition that inequities are due primarily to demand-side factors versus supply-side factors. Even if both are shown to be important, the question remains as to which is the more cost-effective (Handa and Davis 2006).

Two studies have attempted to estimate this in improving schooling enrollment in developing countries (Coady and Parker 2002; Handa 2002). Although no similar health or nutrition study has been undertaken to date, Handa and Davis (2006) noted that health care—particularly preventive health care—differs from education in that asymmetries in information are more acute and poor households may be less likely to seek care due to a lack of information, which would justify government intervention to correct this market failure.[3]

A second assumption is that poor women do not have adequate health education or knowledge. The inclusion of educational health talks as a condition for the cash transfer (mainly targeted toward the women of beneficiary households) is based on this assumption.

The third is that a population needs to be incentivized to make use of health services. By conditioning the transfer on certain types of desired behavior, CCT programs assume that increases in household income from monetary transfers alone will not be enough to induce major changes in human capital investment. This assumption may not hold. There may be a level of transfer that would induce the desired behavior without setting a condition. In that case, the relative cost-effectiveness of a conditioned and nonconditioned transfer scheme should each be calculated. A possible major source of inefficiency in CCT programs is paying people for what they would do in the absence of a payment (Sadoulet, Finan, and de Janvry 2002). Modeling the probability that a given beneficiary will use the conditioned health services under different transfer scenarios is a worthwhile endeavor.

A fourth assumption is that the program will have an effect only if conditionality is monitored and compliance is enforced. Program designers have

3. According to Handa and Davis (2006), "The demand for quality health care is difficult to model because it is hard to measure (and control for) the exogenous price of different alternatives, but there is evidence that both quality and access are also important determinants of utilization."

feared that in the absence of monitoring compliance with the conditions and establishing disincentives for noncompliance (such as docking transfers when conditions are not met), CCT beneficiaries will not comply with program conditions. Two important aspects may counter this assumption. The first is that the mere signaling by the authorities (or program officials) that compliance will be monitored sends the beneficiaries a message stressing the importance of the activity. Second, the presence of conditions implies that there is a risk of losing the transfers.

Schady and Araujo (2006) examine the education component of Ecuador's CCT program, in which beneficiaries were told that compliance would be monitored (but no verification was done). Their findings seem to imply that the mere suggestion of conditionality was sufficient to induce a significant change in the behavior of poor households.[4] Similar work has not yet been done for health. There is also limited knowledge about how long the mere threat of monitoring compliance can substitute for actual compliance.

A fifth assumption in the design of conditional cash transfer programs is that information induces behavioral change. Perhaps by default rather than deliberation, the educational health talks have tended to expose beneficiaries passively to health information. Expecting that such interventions will have an effect assumes that information in and of itself will induce behavior change.

Sixth is the assumption that how CCT resources are allocated within the household depends on who is the official recipient. The transfer, it is argued, should be made to mothers or female caretakers, based on the assumption that they are more likely to invest in the welfare of the children. This assumes, in turn, that the recipient also decides on how the money is used.

Seventh is the assumption that the supply side of services is in place or will follow demand. With the exception of those that include supply-side strengthening, such as RPS in Nicaragua, most CCT programs assume that existing supply-side capacity is adequate to meeting the demand of beneficiaries. If the problem is on the supply side, the thinking goes, then the transfer needs to be made to the supply side, and if the problem is low use of services because beneficiaries do not understand the benefits of preventive care or know

---

4. Schady and Araujo (2006) reported effects on enrollment that are two and a half times as large as those observed in Progresa and attributes this difference to the much lower baseline level of school attendance and enrollment in Ecuador than in Mexico. A similar phenomenon is observed across other impact evaluations; countries that start with lower baselines see larger effects, which may indicate the appropriateness of CCT programs in poorer countries and areas without the need for intensive monitoring of conditionality.

that services are available, then the transfer should be made to the demand side (the beneficiaries). The hope is that governments and providers will increase supply-side inputs if beneficiaries begin to demand services and hold providers accountable.

A reflection on available alternatives to increase use is needed. First, policy-makers should determine whether a budget-constrained government should focus on quantity (increasing use) rather than on quality (improving the effectiveness of existing services to existing users). Second, they should consider whether there are alternative interventions to increase use.

The eighth assumption is that use of (public) health services will improve the health of those receiving the services. By conditioning transfers on the use of preventive services, primarily in public sector clinics, CCT programs clearly assume this to be the case. The assumption relates both to the quality of the services provided and to the quality and effectiveness of substitute products and services.

The ninth assumption is that measured health impacts are those that can be expected to improve and are measured appropriately. This assumption holds if the program addresses the factors that affect both decisions and outcomes. CCTs, for example, target the reduction of infant and maternal mortality. Depending on the context, however, these outcomes may be influenced more by the availability and use of a quality hospital during birth than by maternal nutritional status. In addition, the evaluation instruments used to gauge program effectiveness are assumed to be appropriate to capture the changes that arise because of the intervention. In poor regions, where a significant portion of births occur outside health facilities, the fact that CCT programs evaluate infant and maternal mortality based on facility reports rather than on sample surveys may lead to underestimating mortality measures.

The program effect model—that is, the health change attributable to participation in and compliance with a CCT program—and the underlying assumptions are represented schematically in figure 6-1. The programs in Colombia, Mexico, and Nicaragua modeled the effects that the programs were to have on poverty, inequality, consumption, and school attendance to provide a framework for assessing the results of the evaluations.

Few programs—save those dealing with the demand for health services in Honduras and nutrition effects in Mexico and Nicaragua—have modeled health effects. Although the general omission could be related to the lack of linkages between data sets for some types of outcomes (such as nutritional status or use of specific types of preventive care), in most cases, the health and

Figure 6-1. *Evaluation of Program Impact*

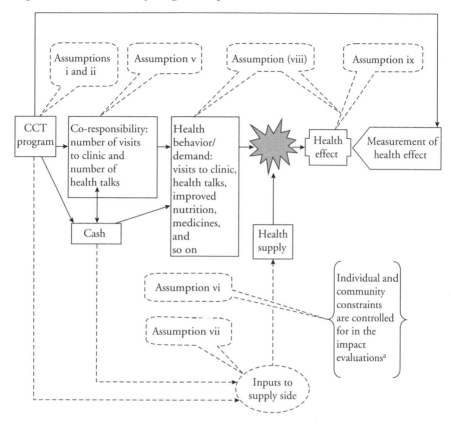

Source: Author.
a. Individual constraints and resources: income, education, information, genetic endowment, preferences, and so on. Community resources and constraints: prices, provider location, disease environment, cultural norms, laws, and the like.

nutrition objectives were essentially afterthoughts not meriting more in-depth analysis.

Design Features

Existing literature provides numerous analyses of the design and implementation features of CCT programs (Handa and Davis 2006; Rawlings and Rubio 2003). We therefore only summarize these findings and present them as basic background information (see box 6-1).

Box 6-1. *The CCT Program Cycle*

The CCT program cycle involves a rough sequence of activities:

—Select program areas (geographic targeting) and coordinate with health and education sectors,
—Identify beneficiary households (household targeting),
—Enroll beneficiaries (involving beneficiary meetings in each community to inform participants of their rights and responsibilities under the program),
—Organize supply responses in advance of generating demand (and supply transfers where relevant),
—Verify conditionality involving the distribution, collection, and processing of clinic and school attendance records,
—Deliver demand transfers (including calculating transfers based on compliance levels, informing beneficiaries about scheduled transfers, and ensuring that the disbursement and payment of transfers through banks or post offices are conducted in a timely and orderly manner), and
—Monitor and evaluate the program internally, including supervision, spot checks, audits, and so on.

Conditions for Payment

To receive transfers each month, households must comply with conditions related to using preventive health services and attending health education sessions. None of these relates explicitly to improved nutrition, but improved nutrition is expected to come as a result of the higher income and greater knowledge about nutrition attained by participants in the program's education and training components.

Conditionality seems to work, although there are few documented studies comparing conditional and unconditional transfers. A comparative impact evaluation by Davis and his colleagues (2002) of Mexico's Progresa program (precursor to Oportunidades) and an unconditioned transfer to poor farmers finds that although overall increases in food consumption were comparable, the effects on health and schooling were significantly greater under Progresa, suggesting that conditionality did make a difference.

Conditions were stated, but compliance was not necessarily monitored. When effective monitoring was in place (Colombia, Mexico, Nicaragua, and Jamaica), compliance was generally extremely high, ranging from 99 percent in Mexico (Behrman and Todd 1999) to 94 percent in Jamaica (Mathematica Policy Research 2005). In cases without monitoring, the evidence was mixed.

In Honduras, for example, women were required to deposit a bar-coded, certified attendance slip in an urn for every required visit to a health center, but no beneficiary was ever suspended for noncompliance (Morris and others 2004). In addition, payments were also irregular and may be responsible for the absence of observed effects. In Ecuador, Schady and Araujo (2006) found that the announcement of conditionality, even if not enforced, was enough to induce a large and significant change in behavior with respect to school attendance. Table 6-1 presents the conditions for payment in each program.

CCT conditions are politically appealing, but administratively challenging and costly to monitor and enforce. Handa and Davis (2006) reported that up to 20 percent of Progresa program costs could be related to enforcing conditionality, raising the issue of whether these costs are worth the added benefits associated with a conditional transfer, given that conditional transfers add value only if the effect on outcomes is significantly greater than that of unconditional transfers.

Transfer Design

Transfers related to health and nutrition conditions are generally lump sum, but in other respects they vary in design. In Colombia, Jamaica, and Mexico, the amount represents the difference between the consumption level of the average extremely poor household and the food poverty line (with some variations). The goal is both basic and political: to move households living in indigence to a minimum level of consumption. In addition, minimum consumption is considered a prerequisite to investing in human capital. Another approach, used in Honduras, is to base the amount of the transfer on the costs of accessing health care.

For this chapter, it is important to note that the lump-sum structure favors smaller families and that the combined amount of the transfer (representing both schooling and health-nutrition subsidies) is what influences the results achieved. On average, payments range from 10 to 25 percent of total consumption among beneficiary households. Table 6-2 summarizes the criteria for determining monthly benefits and the amount of the monthly transfers for each program.

Eligibility and Targeting

Because CCT programs are directed to poor families—generally those with children—a central feature is explicit targeting to determine eligibility for benefits. PRAF and RPS apply geographic targeting strategies only. Poor localities are identified using an index of well-being usually based on census and survey information. Program localities are selected randomly up to a program budget constraint, and all households within the selected localities are eligible to enroll in the program. Progresa and Oportunidades, FA, and Bolsa Familia apply a first

Table 6-1. *Conditions for Payment in CCT Programs*

Country and program	Condition
Brazil (Bolsa Familia)	Children from birth to six years old must have an updated immunization card
	Pregnant and breastfeeding women must make "regular" visits to health centers
	Children from birth to fifteen years of age must make "regular" visits to health centers
Colombia (Familias en Acción)	Children ages birth to four years must attend growth-monitoring visits according to a Ministry of Health protocol (six a year for ages birth to one year, two a year for ages one to three, and one a year for ages three to four)
	Mothers must attend bimonthly health education workshops
Honduras (PRAF)	Children must attend growth-monitoring visits according to Ministry of Health protocol
	Pregnant women must keep at least four prenatal care visits
Jamaica (PATH)	Children ages birth to six must attend checkups every two months during ages birth to one and twice a year thereafter
Mexico (Progresa, Oportunidades)	Children ages birth to twenty-three months must be fully immunized and attend growth-monitoring visits every two months[a]
	Children ages twenty-four to sixty months must attend growth-monitoring visits every four months
	Pregnant women must keep at least four prenatal care visits
	Breastfeeding women must keep at least two postpartum care visits
	Other family members must have physical checkups once a year
	Adult family members must attend health talks (female heads of household every two months; other adults once a year)
Nicaragua (RPS)	Mothers must attend bimonthly health education workshops
	Children ages birth to one year must be up-to-date on their vaccinations (not enforced due to supply failures)
	Children under two years of age must attend monthly growth-monitoring or well-baby visits
	Children between two and five years of age must attend bimonthly medical checkups

Source: Authors.

a. Visits include measurements, nutrition supplements equivalent to 100 percent of the recommended daily allowance for micronutrients and 20 percent for protein, and education for parents on nutritional health and hygiene.

Table 6-2. *Payment Amounts in CCT Programs*

Country and program	Monthly monetary benefit	Average monthly transfer (U.S. dollars)	Average transfer as a percent of poverty line	Percent of pretransfer household consumption
Brazil (Bolsa Familia)	$18 per household; $5 per child (up to three children)	24	12	n.a.
Colombia (FA)	$20 per household; $6 per child of primary school age; $12 per child of secondary school age	50	n.a.	30
Honduras (PRAF)	$4 per household; $5 per child	17	8	10
Jamaica (PATH)	$9 per eligible household member (child, elderly, disabled)	45	16	20
Mexico (Progresa and Oportunidades)	$13 per household; $8–$17 per child of primary school age; $25–$32 per child of secondary school age; $12–$22 per child for school supplies (one-time grant)	20	23	25
Nicaragua (RPS)	$18 per household (additional $9 per household with school-age child); $20 per year per child for supplies	25	18	20

Source: Reprinted with permission from Handa and Davis (2006).
n.a. Not available.

round of geographic targeting followed by direct income testing (proxy means) to identify individual households eligible to participate in the program. Other conditions are sometimes established. For example, the FA program requires that participating municipalities have a bank available within a given geographic reference area as well as an adequate supply of health and education services to meet expected increases in demand.

With the exception of Mexico's Progresa and Oportunidades programs, CCT programs are open exclusively to poor households with young children, school-age children, and pregnant women; all other households do not qualify. Categories of eligible children vary depending on the country's nutrition strategy, which sets certain age groups as targets, establishes the official starting age for school, and determines whether the objective is to create human capital or to balance consumption.

In reviewing the efficiency of different targeting strategies, Coady, Grosh, and Hoddinott (2004) found that although performance in a means test strategy varies significantly based on implementation capacity, these instruments display the best results on errors of inclusion and exclusion and can be cost-effective in specific settings. The Mexican targeting strategy reportedly generated social conflict related to targeting individual households within poor communities (Adato, Coady, and Ruel 2000; Coady 2000).

Individual household targeting also has limitations, which may be important if the program is to serve as a safety net. Selecting households based on determinants of poverty tends to prioritize families with small children and exclude poor ones without small children or with elderly heads. Problems have also been detected around the use of point-specific eligibility cutoffs, which somewhat arbitrarily exclude some households, leading to the adverse community effects observed in the Progresa evaluation. Finally, although individual household targeting can improve program efficiency in more heterogeneous settings, in small, rural, and highly marginalized communities, the Mexican experience suggests that geographic targeting alone is sufficient and that the more precise targeting strategy employed by the program is not cost-effective.[5] Table 6-3 presents the characteristics of beneficiaries in each country studied.

The process of beneficiary requalification varies from country to country. Mexico applies the means test questionnaire to existing and potential beneficiaries on a periodic basis. Colombia and other countries initially set limited terms of eligibility generally associated with the expected duration of available financing, but they have since modified the strategy to one more similar to that of Mexico.

With the exception of Oportunidades (as of 2005), most CCT programs have been scaled up gradually and do not reach the universe of their intended beneficiaries. This approach was adopted to test operational procedures and measure the results of the program using impact evaluation methods, but it also is attributable to budget limitations.

5. There are other motivations for the use of formula-based individual (proxy) means testing, such as the reputation of the program for impartiality and transparency. In Mexico, technical people believed in the transparency and impartiality of the approach, even while beneficiaries complained that they could not understand how eligibility was determined; both are probably important.

Table 6-3. *Characteristics of CCT Beneficiaries*

Country and program	Number of beneficiary households	Proportion poor	Year started
Brazil (Bolsa Familia)	An estimated 2 million–5 million (2004)[a]	n.a.	2003
Colombia (FA)	362,000 (2005)	87 percent poor; 44 percent indigent	2001
Honduras (PRAF)	30,000 (2006)	5 percent extremely poor	2000
Jamaica (PATH)	180,000 (2005)	n.a.	2001
Mexico (Progresa and Oportunidades)	5,000,000 (2006)	100 percent extremely poor	1997
Nicaragua (RPS)	30,000 (2004), now closed	n.a.	2000

Source: Authors.
n.a. Not available.
a. Bolsa Familia's administrative records indicate 5.04 million beneficiaries. Household survey data show approximately 2.09 million beneficiaries (Soares and others 2006). The discrepancy is mostly unexplained, although it is attributed to a period of transition from Bolsa Escola/Alimentação to Bolsa Familia.

Program Costs

Little has been done on the comparative costs of programs (for a review of Progresa, PRAF, and RPS, see Caldés, Coady, and Maluccio 2004). In 2000 Mexico's Progresa cost $41 million. The most recent estimates note that, in most cases, program costs amount to less than 1 percent of gross domestic product (Handa and Davis 2006). In 2004 Brazil used $2.1 billion to cover more than 8 million households, and Mexico used $2.8 billion to cover 5 million. Also in 2004 Colombia used $125 million to cover 400,000 households, and Nicaragua used $6.37 million to cover 22,000. In 2005 Honduras used $25 million to cover more than 400,000 households, and Jamaica used $16 million to cover 220,000.

Operational Arrangements

CCT programs have tended to be implemented by specially created entities linked directly to presidential offices or other semiautonomous units. As such, they are institutionally separate from local governments and line ministries. This seems to have contributed to the rapid pace of implementation observed in most programs, but it also has generated institutional and bureaucratic friction among implementing partners.

Supply Conditions

In some countries, minimum supply conditions have had to be met before implementing the demand-side component. In Colombia, this took the form of a minimum ratio of infrastructure provider to beneficiary and the availability of space
to produce more visits with respect to a standard ratio. In Mexico, minimum
distances to facilities were established. In Honduras and Nicaragua, supply-side
strengthening was built into the program to respond to the pressures associated
with increased demand for services and the possibility that quality might decline
with higher productivity. In both cases, implementing the supply-side components brought substantial delays, which were greater than those associated with an
entirely new program.

Evaluation Results

CCT programs in Latin America include impact evaluation components, which
are unprecedented in the region. This is attributable primarily to four factors:

—As a first implementer, Mexico's Progresa program carried out a state-of-
the-art evaluation that led to extensive documentation and dissemination of
program results, which in turn led to program durability and generated demand
for similar evaluations in countries that followed the Mexican model.

—Because cash transfers as a safety net were relatively new in most countries,
policymakers found it necessary to use other methods, such as in-kind subsidies.

—The rapid expansion of the programs and the size of the beneficiary populations created a need for the evaluations as an accountability tool for government,
and the use of independent evaluators has helped to protect the programs from
charges of politicization.[6]

—The participation of the Inter-American Development Bank and the World
Bank appears to have encouraged the inclusion of impact evaluation, making the
experience particularly interesting to examine in light of low evaluation rates of
other programs.

Objectives and Characteristics

The evaluations sought to confirm the existence of expected impacts, measure the
extent of those impacts, identify unanticipated effects, understand beneficiary and

---

6. However, there is evidence of preelectoral expansions of the beneficiary populations in
Colombia and Mexico, although always applying the same targeting criteria.

stakeholder perceptions of the program, and verify that program benefits were delivered cost-effectively.

To achieve these objectives, the CCT evaluations have either experimental designs (Honduras, Mexico, Nicaragua) or quasi-experimental ones (Colombia, Ecuador, Jamaica), with repeated observations from large samples of households in treatment and control groups gathered in surveys conducted before and after program implementation. In general, the experimental evaluations represent the best attempt to measure the impact of CCT programs given that random assignment limits sample selection bias. Quasi-experimental designs must overcome the selection issue, but when handled carefully they can limit bias. Only rarely can an evaluation estimate impacts for the full population of intended beneficiaries.

The design of the sample for each evaluation determined the type of analysis that could be conducted on the data, and each questionnaire determined what results were measured and reported. In general, difference-in-differences estimates of impacts are reported here unless otherwise noted (for more information on the design and implementation of the evaluations, see IFPRI 2001, 2003; Mathematica Policy Research 2005; Behrman and Todd 1999; Maluccio and Flores 2004; Unión Temporal IFS, Econometría S.A., and SEI 2000). Table 6-4 summarizes the characteristics of the evaluation data by country. Results are reported for only a subset of programs that have completed and reported on at least one postprogram round of data collection: Colombia, Honduras, Mexico, and Nicaragua.

Selected Results

Information currently available in the literature on the health- and nutrition-related outputs and outcomes of the CCT programs includes changes in the use, supply, and quality of services; health knowledge, attitudes, and practice; household consumption; vaccination rates; nutritional status; and changes in morbidity, mortality, and fertility.

USE OF SERVICES

As noted earlier, preventive health care is considered an important input for better child health and is often strongly correlated with family background indicators such as parental education. Thus a major expected output of the CCT programs is to mitigate the advantage of socioeconomic background. All of the programs stipulated the use of preventive health services as a condition for transfers. These indicators were measured by all programs using administrative and household surveys.

Table 6-4. *Summary of Evaluation Data for CCT Programs, by Country*

Characteristic	Mexico	Honduras	Nicaragua	Colombia
Evaluation period	Rural, 1997–99; urban, 2002–03	2000–02	2000–02	2002–03
Targeting level (method)	Locality and household (marginality index)	Locality (priority index)	Municipality (70 with lowest half of first graders)	Locality (meet four criteria) and household
Evaluation design	Rural: experimental; urban: quasi-experimental	Experimental	Experimental	Quasi-experimental
Main evaluation methodology	Difference-in-differences; propensity score matching (urban)	Difference-in-differences	Difference-in-differences	Difference-in-differences; propensity score matching
Sample or panel size	Rural: about 22,000 (about 110,000 households or individuals); urban: 17,201 (76,002 households or individuals)	5,096 (25,777 households or individuals)	1,396 (about 8,500 households or individuals)	10,742 (64,500 households or individuals)

Source: Authors.

As expected, use increased significantly on average among the poor because of the programs. The extent of this increase varied, but use was generally larger in rural areas and among the poorest households. Using evaluation survey data, Gertler and Boyce (2001) suggested that Progresa increased the use of public clinics by 53 percent overall. Some findings on the age distribution of service use are surprising, with effects in some programs more pronounced in the older age group (older than three years). Table 6-5 summarizes program effects.

Although data on the use of general preventive care for children in the Mexican program show little effect, use by households appears to have increased dramatically. Overall, Oportunidades increased the average number of preventive health care visits by members of beneficiary families by 20 percent and reduced the likelihood of hospitalization by 2.5 percent (Gutiérrez and others 2005; Gertler and Boyce 2001). When they were hospitalized, Oportunidades beneficiaries were likely to have a stay that was 1.35 days shorter than that of their

Table 6-5. *Program Effects on Use of Health Services, by Country*[a]

Indicator	Mexico, 1998–2000[b]	Honduras, 2000–02[c]	Nicaragua, 2000–02[d]	Colombia, 2001–03[e]
Public clinic visits for children (reference period)	Rural: for birth to two years old, 1.5 percent decrease; for three to five years old, no impact (last six months)	For birth to three years old, 20.2 percent increase (last thirty days)	For birth to three years old, 11 percent increase (last six months)	For birth to two years old, 30 percent increase; for two to four years old, 50 percent increase (completed age-appropriate visits)
Prenatal care visits (number of visits; details)	Rural: no impact; urban:[f] 6.12 percent increase (four or more; Kessner index)[g]	18.7 percent increase (five or more; last pregnancy)	n.a.	n.a.

Source: Authors.

n.a. Not applicable.

a. Each evaluation's sample design determined the type of analysis that could be conducted on the data. In general, difference-in-differences estimates were used to report the impacts.

b. In Mexico, use was not included in the baseline survey, requiring first-difference estimates of impact. Estimates of impact were conducted using difference-in-differences with clinic-level administrative data available before and after the program. Administrative data confirmed an increase in use in program communities, but these statistics were not disaggregated by age group. For children's use of public clinics, Gertler and Boyce (2001). For prenatal care visits, Prado and others (2004).

c. Impact refers to the household package only (demand-side subsidies only) as reported in Morris and others (2004).

d. Maluccio and Flores (2004).

e. Unión Temporal Institute for Fiscal Studies, Econometría, and Sistemas Especializados de Información (2004).

f. Reference period is 2002–03 for urban areas.

g. Index of care received is determined by the number of visits and the timing of each visit; does not include any measure of quality of care received at each visit (Prado and others 2004).

counterparts. Although these analyses have not yet clarified whether decreases in hospitalization are attributable to more or better preventive services or to the effects of better knowledge along with the overall increase in preventive care, it appears that the program is successful in reducing the frequency and severity of morbidity.

Although CCT evaluations assess changes in beneficiary care-seeking practices with respect to total number of visits, particularly well-child visits, the analyses published to date provide only limited information on some of the assumptions and causal pathways. This limits the interpretation of the findings.

First, the motivation for increased use of services may be related to program conditionality, but it could also be attributable to any number of the factors that the programs influence.

Second, net increases in use remain difficult to measure given that some programs, such as those in Colombia and Honduras, do not report on what happens in the private sector. In addition, Mexico's Oportunidades yields no effects on use among the youngest age groups.

Third, the age patterns of changes in use remain difficult to interpret. Some hypotheses on this phenomenon have been offered, but better exploration of the relationship between patterns of use by age and decreases in morbidity and mortality would help to disentangle which parts of the CCT health package influence impact and whether there is a link between service use and health outcomes.

Fourth, although the increases observed in preventive care visits are inherently positive, it is also possible that above a certain number of visits, nonbeneficiary clients may be crowded out or the quality of service may drop. Understanding what the social and individual optimal levels of use are will strengthen future program design.

KNOWLEDGE, ATTITUDES, AND PRACTICE

Health education components are included in all programs, but evaluations have generally not measured health knowledge and attitudes directly. There are, though, a few exceptions. In Mexico, Progresa evaluators have found an increase in dietary quality and calorie consumption. After controlling for the income effect associated with increased calorie consumption, the increase in consumption of more diverse, high nutritional quality foods such as fruits, vegetables, and animal products indicates a possible effect of the nutritional education provided through health education talks (Hoddinott, Skoufias, and Washburn 2000). Prado and his colleagues (2004) reported both increased knowledge of family planning methods in both urban and rural areas and higher use of modern family planning methods in rural areas among program beneficiaries than in the control group.

Evaluators found that Colombia's FA program not only increased the time that children are breastfed but also improved the quality of food consumed by children, increasing the average number of days per week that various proteins, grains, and fruits and vegetables are consumed. The program also increased overall household consumption of high-quality foods (Unión Temporal IFS, Econometría S.A., and SEI 2004).

CONSUMPTION

CCT beneficiary communities and households were, for the most part, poor or extremely poor before the start of the program. The extremely poor, by definition, do not have enough household income to buy basic foodstuffs. In addition to improved quality of foods consumed, increased food consumption is considered the vehicle for achieving improved nutritional status, which is linked to better cognitive and social development, higher levels of educational attainment, and other outcomes. Table 6-6 summarizes program effects on household consumption.

In Mexico, Hoddinott, Skoufias, and Washburn (2000) found that mean household consumption increased significantly among Progresa beneficiary households, a difference of almost 11 percent, and that this effect was more pronounced among the poor.

Table 6-6. *Program Effects on Household Consumption*[a]

Indicator	Mexico, 1997–99[b]	Honduras, 2000–02[c]	Nicaragua, 2000–02[d]	Colombia, 2000–03[e]
Mean per capita food consumption and expenditures	10.6 percent increase	No impact	21 percent increase	20.4 percent increase in urban areas; 22.5 percent increase in rural areas (household total)
Mean per capita total consumption and expenditures	n.a.	No impact	13 percent increase	13.9 percent increase in urban areas; 16.9 percent increase in rural areas (household total)

Source: Authors.
n.a. Not available.

a. Difference-in-differences estimates are reported for Nicaragua, Colombia, and Honduras for food expenditures. Cross-sectional estimates (first difference) are reported for Mexico and total expenditures for Honduras. In Mexico, no consumption data were collected at baseline; in Honduras, a difference in the seasonality of the baseline survey across the control and treatment groups affected baseline nonfood expenditures.

b. Hoddinott, Skoufias, and Washburn (2000).

c. Impact refers to the household package only (demand-side subsidies only), as reported in Morris and others (2004).

d. Maluccio and Flores (2004).

e. Unión Temporal Institute for Fiscal Studies, Econometría, and Sistemas Especializados de Información (2004); estimates are reported for difference-in-differences between treatment group without payment and control group and converted to percentages from the log-point estimates.

In Nicaragua's RPS program in 2002, the average effect on per capita annual household expenditures was about 13 percent of the value before the program. The effect was much larger for extremely poor households than for the nonpoor: 40 and 6 percent of initial per capita expenditures, respectively (Maluccio and Flores 2004). RPS evaluators also reported increases in per capita annual food expenditures, reflecting that most of the additional income supplied by the transfer was put toward the purchase of foodstuffs.

In Colombia, the FA program was found to have increased total consumption, consumption of food, and expenditures on children's clothing in both rural and urban areas, as well as expenditures and consumption on schooling in urban areas. Again, the increased consumption was concentrated among high-quality foods.

Thus, with the exception of the Honduran program, the effect of the program on total household consumption was large and significant, but not surprising. More important, the effects on food consumption and diet diversity were significant. The results of this increased caloric quality are evident in some of the nutritional outcomes described.

SUPPLY

The CCT program effect model includes two main assumptions related to the supply of health services: (a) the current supply of health services is adequate or an increase in services will follow the increase in demand resulting from the program and (b) use will improve health status (assuming that the quality of care available is enough to result in positive changes in health). Little documentation is available on how the programs have affected the availability and quality of health care services or on how supply-side components of the program have affected the observed outcomes.

Using administrative data, Gertler and Boyce (2001) recorded substantially increased numbers of visits in Progresa localities. Qualitative studies also confirmed increased workloads. In an urban setting, medical staff in beneficiary communities reported 23 to 87 percent more visits (Escobar-Latapí and González de la Rocha 2005), and a focus group of health directors reported staff shortages, saturation of services, and lack of supplies (Meneses and others 2005).

The Mexican social development ministry, SEDESOL, reported an increase in the number of health clinics in program localities and in public budgets for health. Escobar-Latapí and González de la Rocha (2005) reported that urban clinics were built in program areas after the program was introduced and included higher salaries for staff, both of which may indicate a supply response to the program.

The Nicaraguan RPS program financed a scale-up of health supply through contracted nongovernmental organization (NGO) providers. Regalía and Castro

(2006) discussed the related increase in the number of health care facilities, but not quality issues or the effect of the health lectures on health-related behaviors and knowledge. Although dedicated funding for increases in health care facilities, staff, training, equipment, and supplies should translate into improvements in these areas, delays in implementation (in training, hiring, and resource transfers) could result in deviations between planned and actual changes. Thus it is not a trivial exercise to evaluate how well and how quickly the supply-side resource transfers are executed. At this point, researchers have been unable to separate the effects of the various components of the program, especially the differences between impacts attributable to the cash transfers and those attributable to supply-side improvements.

QUALITY

Quality of services makes the condition of requiring health center visits meaningful: without adequate quality, expected effects will not occur. Because most of the data on quality come from small-scale and qualitative studies, findings cannot be generalized. The few existing studies pertain to Mexico. In spite of these caveats, it is worth noting that although the number of procedures is higher among beneficiaries, the results of the interventions are not encouraging, suggesting that a priority is to strengthen the quality of care.

In Mexico, the availability and quality of medicines appear to be a major issue. A small-scale facility survey found that public health clinics in a group of Oportunidades localities did not have enough medicines to treat the increased number of patients (Escobar-Latapí and González de la Rocha 2002). Beneficiaries reported that the medicines provided by the public clinics were of inferior quality and that many beneficiaries were choosing more expensive higher-quality drugs at private pharmacies. Neufeld and her colleagues (2005) noted that delivery of nutritional supplements to program localities in Mexico was sometimes delayed, resulting in inadequate supply and potentially reducing the frequency of consumption.

In Colombia, the FA impact evaluation included a health facility survey that collected information about various characteristics related to access and quality of care. The surveys collected information about the hours of operation, types of services offered, number of various services provided in the past year, number and type of current staff, stocks of various medicines, interruptions in service due to labor problems, political unrest, or natural disasters, the previous year's budget and revenue, main sources of revenue, participation in and training received for the program, and other details related to the program. However, the sampling method of facilities is not clear, and this information was not studied or included in the impact evaluation.

VACCINATION RATES

Although vaccination was a condition for transfers in Honduras and Nicaragua, it was not monitored by the program; only the visit was recorded. As a result, estimates of the impact on vaccination rates came from external evaluation of the programs.

The overall contribution of CCT to vaccination coverage appears marginal. In spite of apparent program-attributable increases during a pilot implemented during 2000 and 2001, the Nicaraguan RPS program produced an insignificant average net increase of 6.1 percentage points in up-to-date vaccination levels between 2000 and 2002 (Maluccio and Flores 2004).[7] In Honduras, the PRAF showed marginally higher rates of diphtheria, tetanus, pertussis (DTP)/Pentavalent for children, but insignificant and small differences for maternal mortality (Morris and others 2004). The Colombian program measured DTP prevalence and found an insignificant difference between program participants and controls (Unión Temporal IFS, Econometría, and SEI 2004).

Vaccination is difficult to impose as a condition because it depends on supply. Unlike growth-monitoring visits, if vaccines are not in stock, vaccination cannot occur. The Honduras experience, where supply was variable, is an example of this phenomenon, and results may relate more to the availability of vaccines at health centers than to a demand effect. However, an indirect effect of the program may be that coordination with the Ministry of Health in program areas may in fact generate more supply of the vaccine (Maluccio and Flores 2004).

NUTRITIONAL STATUS

Unlike the unambiguously positive results for food consumption, outcome measures of nutritional status show mixed results. All programs except in Honduras achieved a significant reduction in stunting. Results for the proportion underweight were less consistent: Nicaragua showed a large and significant decline, and Colombia showed an impact only in rural areas for three- to seven-year-olds. No effects on anemia were observed. Table 6-7 summarizes these program effects on

---

7. Maluccio and Flores (2004) included an interesting footnote regarding the quality of administrative data on vaccination that will be relevant to other payment-for-performance schemes; they found that survey reports are substantially lower than the 100 percent recorded in administrative data. The errors may go in both directions.

Table 6-7. *Program Effects on Nutritional Status*

Outcomes	Mexico		Honduras, 2000–02	Nicaragua, 2000–02	Colombia, 2001–03
	1997–99[a]	1997–2003[b]			
Proportion stunted; height-for-age (haz) ≤ −2.0	1997–99: a statistically significant decrease from a baseline of 44 percent (point estimate not reported)	1997–2003: for 2 to six years old, 29 percent decrease for girls, 11 percent decrease for boys	For birth to four years old, no impact	For birth to four years old, 5.5 percentage point decrease	For birth to two years old, 6.9 percentage point decrease; for 2 to 6 years, no impact
Proportion under weight; weight-for-age (waz) ≤ −2.0	No impact	No impact	For birth to four years old, no impact	For birth to four years old, 6 percentage point decrease	For rural, no impact for birth to three years old; 3.4 percentage point decrease for three to seven years old; for urban: no impact
Anemia (prevalence)	No impact	3 percent decrease	For twelve to twenty-three months old, no impact	For six to fifty-nine months old, no impact	Not measured

Source: Authors.

a. Stunting, underweight, and anemia (Behrman and Hoddinott 2000); data collected by Instituto Nacional de Salud Pública 1998 and 1999 were then matched to the evaluation data collected by Progresa.

b. Gertler and Fernald (2004).

nutritional status. A recent paper, however, showed that a doubling of cash transfers in Oportunidades resulted in a highly significant increase in the height-for-age Z score of 0.20 and a reduction in the proportion of stunting of −0.10 (Fernald, Gertler, and Neufeld 2008).

MORBIDITY

Measured morbidity may increase or decrease as a result of the CCT intervention. On the one hand, more preventive care and health knowledge may lead to fewer episodes of illness. On the other hand, higher levels of health knowledge and more frequent visits to health centers may increase the probability that mothers will diagnose illnesses more frequently or more accurately and will seek care when it is required. Moreover, improved health may lead to increased recognition of the symptoms of morbidity, such as respiratory infections, and thus increase the demand for curative care (Oppenheimer 2001). These hypotheses have rarely been explored by the evaluations, but where they have been measured (mainly in Mexico), CCT appears to decrease the incidence and prevalence of morbidity.

The evaluation of Mexico's program found that the program had a negative and statistically significant impact on the probability of child illness for all age groups, but not until a child had been receiving benefits for at least twelve months (Gertler and Boyce 2001). In rural areas a small decrease in sick days was observed only for the productive-age population, whereas a larger effect and wider age range was seen in urban areas. Overall, the number of days lost to illness decreased by 20 percent among beneficiary families (Gutiérrez and others 2005).

An Oportunidades study of the effect of the program on indigenous populations found that the program decreased illness rates from 0.2 to 3.5 percent, with the greatest effects observed among children under three years old (Quiñones 2006). The average estimated program effect differed substantially from Gertler's findings, most likely because of differences in sampling size and approach used. Positive program effects observed for indigenous beneficiaries were similar to those for nonindigenous beneficiaries. On the one hand, this finding could be considered a weakness of the program, as Quiñones argued, given the implicit assumption that the average effect of the program should be larger on poorer and more marginalized groups. On the other hand, it is remarkable that the benefits were equivalent for both groups when one takes into account evidence that indigenous groups have a more difficult time complying with CCT conditions because of language and cultural barriers.

With respect to chronic disease–related morbidity, the required regular checkups and participation in health talks may have a positive effect on household and social norms related to food intake and activity. However, the income transfer to the household could make more affordable some behaviors that increase the risk of chronic diseases (for example, the consumption of junk foods, soft drinks, and alcohol). The single study on this issue from Mexico found encouraging results. Fernald, Gertler, and Olaiz (2005) found that the baseline prevalence of obesity (24 percent), hypertension (39 percent), and diabetes (19 percent) was high among the rural poor in Mexico and that participation in Oportunidades significantly reduced the prevalence of all except diabetes. Symptoms of hypertension and diabetes were also significantly reduced via participation in the program.

These results suggest that if a CCT is implemented to achieve health objectives in countries well into the epidemiological transition, requiring poor adults to seek preventive care and checkups may be an effective strategy.

MORTALITY

Mortality was not measured directly by the evaluations. Only the Mexican program used administrative data to analyze program effects. Although infant and maternal mortality were found to have declined significantly in program areas, the reliance on administrative data, particularly in the case of maternal mortality, is problematic.

Hernández and his colleagues (2003) examined the impact of Oportunidades on maternal and infant mortality using data for the period from 1995 to 2002 from the Ministry of Health and the National Institute of Statistics, Geography, and Information Technology. For the entire period, maternal mortality was 11 percent lower in the municipalities with at least one locality incorporated in the Oportunidades program. For the entire period from 1997 to 2003, infant mortality was 2 percent lower in the municipalities incorporated in Oportunidades than in the nonincorporated ones. Estimates of absolute numbers indicate that, thanks to the program, 340 infant deaths a year, on average, were avoided during this period. The impact of Oportunidades on infant mortality at the municipal level increased relative to the proportion of the population participating in the program.

FERTILITY

Although the literature on financial incentives in fertility suggests that fertility is declining throughout the developing world and that welfare programs and state policies have not been enough to generate a positive fertility response, some are concerned that fertility levels might be adversely affected by CCT programs. Data from Colombia, Mexico, and Nicaragua indicate that fertility rates decreased in the presence of the program, but the Honduras program, which applied a different payment incentive structure, observed an increase in fertility.

Stecklov and his colleagues (2006) examined the unintended effects of CCT programs in Honduras, Mexico, and Nicaragua on fertility levels and found that unintentional incentives for childbearing in Honduras (a health-nutrition subsidy that is not lump sum and varies by number of children and pregnant women in a beneficiary household) may have contributed to a 2 to 4 percentage point increase in fertility. This effect (which was not observed in Mexico and Nicaragua, where health and nutrition grants are lump sum) may be related to an increase in marriage rates, the effects of the program on the presence of the partner, or a temporary response to the program's unintended incentives.

Prado and others (2004) found that in rural areas in the Oportunidades program the proportion of women using family planning methods decreased in both intervention and control localities. The average number of children per woman of reproductive age also decreased in both groups. The evaluation of Colombia's FA found a relatively large decline in fertility between baseline and follow-up surveys (among control and intervention groups), but did not explore the reasons behind these changes.

Limitations

The CCT program evaluations set a high standard for impact evaluation, but major limitations are related to the sampling designs and construction of counterfactual groups. With respect to health in particular, the limitations relate to the use of instruments and questions for studying the relationship between specific components of the program and specific outputs or outcomes.

Evaluations have paid minimal attention to the impact on health-related behaviors, attitudes, and household decisionmaking or how these factors contribute to or limit impacts on outcomes. The majority of the program evaluations have focused instead on the effects on specific outcomes of health indicators (such as incidences of illnesses, child growth) and outputs (such as use rates of public facilities for preventative, curative, and prenatal care).

Improvements in these outcomes and outputs were listed as goals, so determining the program's impact is an important first step. But because many of the outputs—especially the use of preventive and prenatal care—are conditions for transfers, the program should lead to increases. Furthermore, outcomes such as illnesses and child growth are observed more or less at the end of a black box, and evaluations are little help in understanding exactly how the program operates to bring about such changes in outcomes.

Both Oportunidades and RPS were found to have improved health outcomes among young children, for example, but it is not clear exactly which components were important to the improvements. The impacts could be attributable to the receipt of nutritional supplements, increased use of preventative and prenatal care services, increased food consumption, increased knowledge in topics covered by the health information lectures (such as proper hygiene and food preparation, best practices for breastfeeding, and treatment of diarrhea), or even increased coverage and timeliness of vaccinations. Understanding the role of such factors in influencing outcomes is critical to developing more effective programs.

Finally, although the program's rationale and effect model indicate that the reduction of out-of-pocket and opportunity costs associated with seeking health care is both the principal mechanism to increase use and one of the outcome variables, one would expect to observe impact. No evaluation has analyzed these aspects.

Conclusions

CCT impact evaluations provided unambiguous evidence that financial incentives increase the poor's use of key services. Further, the evaluations indicated that cash transfers, accompanied by information, social support, weight monitoring, and micronutrient supplementation, can stimulate healthier feeding practices and dramatically improve young children's nutritional status, particularly the incidence of stunting. The Mexican program suggests that adult health may also benefit.

The numerous dimensions of CCT program benefits are an added attraction. Unlike specific demand-side incentives, CCT programs recognize that the barriers to better health and service use are part of a larger problem: scarcity of household resources. Findings suggest that the poorest households must reach a minimum threshold of food consumption before they are able to make other investments in their well-being. Further, better nutritional status improves the effectiveness of health treatments. What is more, the gains associated with both preventive care and schooling are irreversible.

The mixed picture with respect to outcomes—vaccination, nutritional status, and (where there are data) morbidity and mortality—suggest that assumptions might not be accurate and thus that our expectations for impacts may be incorrect.

Financial incentives are a blunt instrument that can have many unintended effects, such as those observed on fertility in Honduras. For this reason, it is important to design incentives carefully. This is particularly important with respect to the health and nutrition components, because the evidence reviewed seems to indicate that these aspects of the programs have been underdesigned.

Several key issues need to be addressed when designing CCT programs. Three are particularly important. One is identifying the marginal benefit of conditioned versus unconditioned transfers. Monitoring conditionality is costly, and it is important to determine whether conditions are necessary and, if so, whether enforcement is critical. A second consideration is the baseline status of outcomes. A low baseline means that a CCT program may be able to achieve better results; a higher baseline means that a CCT program may not have any impact or may not be cost-effective. The third issue is the relative cost-effectiveness of investing in the supply side rather than the demand side of the health system. Supply and demand are jointly determined. Although paying poor households to use preventive services does help to increase use, what happens at the health post is still unclear. If quality declines, or nonbeneficiaries are crowded out, the programs may pay too much for the care that beneficiaries receive. In other words, negative spillovers in service quality from demand-side programs may be greater than the net gain to beneficiaries. Higher demand, however, can encourage improvements in efficiency and quality.

Each of these issues centers on the need to assess the supply side and model the demand for health care before finalizing program design. Cost-effectiveness should also be considered with respect to nutrition: program designers must assess how well a CCT program performs relative to an in-kind transfer or food price subsidy. The effects on use, consumption, and nutrition also should be modeled to determine the burden of conditioned services for an average household.

A final word on evaluation: we have found limited analysis on the health effects of CCT programs outside of Mexico, and even less on the impact of programs on health providers. Expanding the scope of future CCT program impact evaluations to include effects on outputs such as knowledge, behaviors, service access, and service supply can help to improve our understanding of how the program works to achieve improvements.

However, the choice to expand questionnaires or add instruments most likely involves a trade-off of depth in other areas to maintain data quality. Many of the program evaluation surveys already include questions that could be used to expand the scope of impact evaluations (such as the facility surveys and mother's health knowledge collected for FA), yet the data have not been used. Perhaps giving more researchers access to the data will lead to further studies, the results of which could be used to guide the development and design of future evaluations and instruments.

Probably one of the largest gaps in the impact evaluations discussed is the lack of information about the supply of health care services. The quality and quantity of health care available to poor households could have a large effect on the health status of parents as well as children. Improving the tools and strategies used to measure the quality of service delivery was the topic of a 2006 World Bank workshop, in which participants shared their experiences in collecting and studying a variety of aspects related to the provision of health care services. One of the most common observations was that matching facility-level data on supply and quality to household-level data on health outcomes improved their use. CCT program impact evaluations thus appear to be the most appropriate setting in which to use supply-side instruments and develop approaches for studying the relationship between demand and supply factors of health outcomes.

Taking these factors into account during the design of a CCT program provides a unique and important opportunity to improve the effectiveness of these programs and, given the targeting to the poor, the effectiveness of the health system itself on health and nutrition status (see box 6-2).

Box 6-2. *Designing and Evaluating a CCT*

Design and evaluation encompass the following steps:

—*Check whether assumptions hold.* Using existing data, a baseline evaluation survey, or both, assess whether the underlying assumptions of the CCT model hold for the country in which you are working. For example, do the poor underutilize preventive services? What is the principal barrier to access? For instance, are rates of oral rehydration therapy use low primarily because procurement and distribution systems are weak or because the poor face high costs associated with seeking care?

—*Model program effects beforehand.* Model the effects of a transfer in the design phase and set the amount of the transfer based on the effects you want to achieve.

—*Assess the supply situation and design conditions carefully.* Conditions must be just right: not too burdensome, yet not irrelevant. Forcing use of poor-quality primary health clinics in the public sector may not produce the desired results, so where quality is a problem, contract out services for beneficiaries; deal with the health sector implications later.

(continued)

Box 6-2. *Designing and Evaluating a CCT (continued)*

—*Decide whether to enforce compliance, but always evaluate compliance.* Put the information system requirements in place that are necessary to enforce compliance (or decide not to enforce compliance) and evaluate what happens.
—*Target the extremely poor.* Because program effects are most pronounced when directed toward households with the poorest outcomes, it is critical to target the extremely poor, using the most cost-effective targeting method for a given setting.
—*Learn from other programs.* Multilateral development banks and donors should ensure that evaluations and experienced staff are made available to support governments in the development of programs. Refer to existing literature in planning and implementing programs.

References

Adato, Michelle, David Coady, and Marie Ruel. 2000. "An Operations Evaluation of Progresa from the Perspective of Beneficiaries, Promotoras, School Directors, and Health Staff." Washington: International Food Policy Research Institute.

Behrman, Jere R., and John Hoddinott. 2000. "An Evaluation of the Impact of Progresa on Preschool Child Height." Washington: International Food Policy Research Institute.

Behrman, Jere R., and Petra E. Todd. 1999. "A Report on the Sample Sizes Used for the Evaluation of the Education, Health, and Nutrition Program (Progresa) of Mexico." Washington: International Food Policy Research Institute.

Caldés, Natalia, David Coady, and John A. Maluccio. 2004. *The Cost of Poverty Alleviation Transfer Programs: A Comparative Analysis of Three Programs in Latin America.* IFPRI Discussion Paper 174. Washington: International Food Policy Research Institute.

Coady, David. 2000. "The Application of Social Cost-Benefit Analysis to the Evaluation of Progresa." Washington: International Food Policy Research Institute (December).

Coady, David, Margaret Grosh, and John Hoddinott. 2004. *The Targeting of Transfers in Developing Countries: Review of Experience and Lessons.* Washington: World Bank.

Coady, David, and Susan W. Parker. 2002. "A Cost-effectiveness Analysis of Demand- and Supply-side Interventions: The Case of PROGRESA in Mexico." IFPRI Discussion Paper 127. Washington: International Food Policy Research Institute.

Davis, Benjamin, Sudhanshu Handa, M. Ruiz Arranz, M. Stampini, and Paul Winters. 2002. "Conditionality and the Impact of Program Design on Household Welfare: Comparing Two Diverse Cash Transfer Programs in Rural Mexico." ESA Working Paper 02-10. New York: United Nations, Food and Agricultural Organization.

Eichler, Rena. 2006. "Can 'Pay for Performance' Increase Utilization by the Poor and Improve the Quality of Health Services?" Discussion paper for the first meeting of the Working Group on Performance-Based Incentives. Washington: Center for Global Development.

Ensor, Tim, and Stephanie Cooper. 2004 "Overcoming Barriers to Health Service Access: Influencing the Demand Side." *Health Policy and Planning* 19 (2): 69–79.

Escobar-Latapí, Agustín, and Mercedes González de la Rocha. 2002. "Evaluación cualitativa del programa de desarrollo humano Oportunidades, seguimiento de impacto, 2001–2002, comunidades de 2,500 a 50,000 habitantes: Evaluación de resultados de impacto del programa de desarrollo humano Oportunidades." Mexico City: Centro de Investigaciones y Estudios Superiores en Antropología Social (December).

———. 2005. "Evaluación cualitativa del programa Oportunidades en zonas urbanas, 2003." In *Evaluación externa de impacto del Programa Oportunidades 2003,* edited by Bernardo Hernández Prado and Mauricio Hernández Ávila. Mexico City: Instituto Nacional de Salud Pública, Centro de Investigaciones y Estudios Superiores en Antropología Social.

Fernald, Lia, Paul Gertler, and Lynnette Neufeld. 2008. "Role of Cash in Conditional Cash Transfer Programmes for Child Health, Growth, and Development: An Analysis of Mexico's *Oportunidades.*" *Lancet* 371 (9615): 789–91.

Fernald, Lia, Paul Gertler, and Gustavo Olaiz. 2005. "Impacto de mediano plazo del Programa Oportunidades sobre la obesidad y las enfermedades crónicas en áreas rurales." In *Evaluación externa de impacto del Programa Oportunidades 2004,* edited by Bernardo Hernández Prado and Mauricio Hernández Ávila. Cuernavaca, Mexico: Instituto Nacional de Salud Pública.

Gertler, Paul, and Simone Boyce. 2001. "An Experiment in Incentive-Based Welfare: The Impact of Progresa on Health in Mexico." London: Royal Economic Society.

Gertler, Paul, and Lia Fernald. 2004. "The Medium-Term Impact of Oportunidades on Child Development in Rural Areas." Washington: World Bank.

Grossman, Michael 1972. "On the Concept of Health Capital and the Demand for Health." *Journal of Political Economy* 80 (2): 223–55.

Gutiérrez, Juan Pablo, Sergio Bautista, Paul Gertler, Mauricio Hernández, and Stefano M. Bertozzi. 2005. "Impacto de Oportunidades en la morbilidad y el estado de salud de la población beneficiaria y en la utilización de los servicios de salud. Resultados de corto plazo en zonas urbanas y de mediano plazo en zonas rurales." In *Evaluación externa del impacto del programa Oportunidades 2004,* edited by Bernardo Hernández Prado and Mauricio Hernández Ávila. Mexico City: Instituto Nacional de Salud Pública, Centro de Investigaciones y Estudios Superiores en Antropología Social.

Handa, Sudhanshu. 2002. "Raising Primary School Enrollment in Developing Countries: The Relative Importance of Supply and Demand." *Journal of Development Economics* 69 (1): 103–28.

Handa, Sudhanshu, and Benjamin Davis. 2006. "The Experience of Conditional Cash Transfers in Latin America and the Caribbean." *Development Policy Review* 24 (5): 513–36.

Hernández, Bernardo, J. E. Urquieta, F. Meneses, M. C. Baltazar, and M. Hernández. 2003. "Evaluación del cumplimiento de metas, costos unitarios y apego del programa Oportunidades a las reglas de operación: Evaluación de resultados de impacto del programa de desarrollo humano Oportunidades." Mexico City: Instituto Nacional de Salud Público.

Hoddinott, John, Emmanuel Skoufias, and Ryan Washburn. 2000. "The Impact of Progresa on Consumption: A Final Report." Washington: International Food Policy Research Institute (September).

IFPRI (International Food Policy Research Institute). 2001. "Informe: Sistema de evaluación de la fase piloto de la Red de Protección Social de Nicaragua." Washington.

————. 2003. "Sexto informe: Proyecto PRAF/BID fase II; Impacto intermedio." Washington.

Maluccio, John A., and Rafael Flores. 2004. *Impact Evaluation of a Conditional Cash Transfer Program: The Nicaraguan Red de Protección Social.* Food Consumption and Nutrition Division Discussion Paper 184. Washington: International Food Policy Research Institute.

Mathematica Policy Research. 2005. "Evaluation of Jamaica's PATH Program: Interim Report." Princeton, N.J.

Meneses G., Fernando, and others. 2005. "Evaluación del cumplimiento de las metas, los costos unitarios y el apego del programa a las reglas de operación 2004." In *Evaluación externa del impacto del programa Oportunidades 2004: Aspectos económicos y sociales,* edited by Bernardo Hernández Prado and Mauricio Hernández Ávila. Mexico City: Instituto Nacional de Salud Pública, Centro de Investigaciones y Estudios Superiores en Antropología Social.

Morris, Saul S., R. Flores, P. Olinto, and J. M. Medina. 2004. "Monetary Incentives in Primary Health Care and Effects on Use and Coverage of Preventive Health Care Interventions in Rural Honduras: Cluster Randomised Trial." *Lancet* 364 (9450): 2030–37.

Mushkin, Selma J. 1962. "Health as an Investment." *Journal of Political Economy* 70 (5): 129–57.

Neufeld, Lynnette, Daniela Sotres Alvarez, Lourdes Flores López, Lizbeth Tolentino Mayo, Jorge Jiménez Ruiz, and Juan Rivera Dommarco. 2005. "A Study of the Consumption of the Food Supplements Nutrisano and Nutrivida by Children and Women Beneficiaries of Oportunidades in Urban Areas." External evaluation of the impact of the human development program Oportunidades. Mexico City: Instituto Nacional de Salud Pública.

Oppenheimer, Stephen J. 2001. "Iron and Its Relation to Immunity and Infectious Disease." *Journal of Nutrition* 131 (2): S616–35.

Prado, Bernardo, José Urquieta Salomón, María Ramírez Villalobos, and José Luis Figueroa. 2004. "Impacto de Oportunidades en la salud reproductiva de la población beneficiaria." Mexico City: Instituto Nacional de Salud Pública de México.

Quiñones, Esteban J. 2006. "The Indigenous Heterogeneity of Oportunidades: Ample or Insufficient Human Capital Accumulation?" Unpublished manuscript. Washington: International Food Policy Research Institute, Development Strategy and Governance Division.

Rawlings, Laura B., and G. M. Rubio. 2003. "Evaluating the Impact of Conditional Cash Transfer Programs: Lessons from Latin America." Washington: World Bank.

Regalía, Ferdinando, and Leslie Castro. 2006. "Health Interventions in the Nicaraguan Red de Protección Social." Washington: Center for Global Development.

Sadoulet, Elisabeth, Frederico Finan, and Alain de Janvry. 2002. "Decomposing the Channels of Influence of Conditional Transfers in a Structural Model of Educational Choice." Berkeley: University of California.

Schady, Norbert, and María Caridad Araujo. 2006. "Cash Transfers, Conditions, School Enrollment, and Child Work: Evidence from a Randomized Experiment in Ecuador." Impact Evaluation Series 3, World Bank Policy Research Working Paper 3930. Washington: World Bank.

Soares, Fabio Veras, and others. 2006. "Cash Transfer Programmes in Brazil: Impacts on Inequality and Poverty." International Poverty Centre Working Paper 21. Brasilia: United Nations Development Programme.

Stecklov, Guy, Paul Winters, Jessica Todd, and Ferdinando Regalía. 2006. "Demographic
   Externalities from Poverty Programs in Developing Countries: Experimental Evidence from
   Latin America." Department of Economics Working Paper 2006-1. Washington: American
   University.
Unión Temporal Institute for Fiscal Studies, Econometría S.A., and Sistemas Especializados
   de Información. 2000. *Evaluación del impacto del programa de Familias en Acción: Informe
   metodológico.* Bogotá: DAPR-FIP (Departamento Administrativo de la Presidencia de
   la República, Fondo de Inversión para la Paz) and DNP (Departamento Nacional de
   Planeamiento).
————. 2004. *Evaluación del impacto del programa Familias en Acción: Informe del primer
   seguimiento.* Bogotá: DAPR-FIP (Departamento Administrativo de la Presidencia de
   la República, Fondo de Inversión para la Paz) and DNP (Departamento Nacional de
   Planeamiento).

7

United States: Orienting Pay-for-Performance to Patients

Kevin Volpp and Mark Pauly

Highlights

Evidence from randomized controlled trials in the United States suggests that demand-side performance incentives have increased follow-up rates of patients wanting to learn the results of screening tests and take treatments requiring limited changes in behavior.

For interventions that require more than time-limited changes in behavior (such as smoking cessation), incentives may attract people to begin treatment, but as of yet there is scant evidence as to whether success rates are sustained once extrinsic rewards cease.

Experience and evidence from developed countries suggest that patient-targeted performance incentives may be especially effective in developing countries where financial obstacles are great, and additional income is highly valued.

The term *pay for performance* in the United States has become synonymous with supply-side incentives focused on providers, with the goal of improving the quality of care delivered by clinicians, hospitals, and health care systems. Relatively little attention has been paid to demand-side approaches to modifying health behavior.

The focus on supply-side approaches within the United States is striking because smoking, diet, sedentary lifestyles, and other individual behaviors account for a substantial portion of all health care costs and cause hundreds of thousands of deaths annually within the United States (DiMatteo 2004; Mokdad and others 2004). Although smoking is the leading cause of preventable mortality and accounts for approximately 435,000 deaths each year (Mokdad and others 2004), only 2 to 3 percent of smokers quit each year (Bartlett and others 1994; Hughes 2003). Poor control of blood pressure—the principal modifiable risk factor for stroke (SHEP, Cooperative Research Group 1991; Amery and others 1985), coronary heart disease, congestive heart failure, and end-stage renal disease (Klag and others 1996; American Heart Association 2002)—is seen in approximately 70 percent of the 50 million Americans who have hypertension (Klag and others 1996; McDonald, Garg, and Haynes 2002), and failure to adhere to medications is a common cause of poor control (Monane and others 1996; Eisen and others 1990; Nelson and others 1980). Reducing these and other preventable causes of morbidity and mortality depends on more effective strategies for changing health-related behavior.

Performance-based incentives targeted at patients might be particularly helpful in improving health in developing countries for a number of reasons. Far more medical expenditures are paid out of pocket in developing countries. In the United States the proportion is 13 percent—a stark contrast to the 38 to 84 percent in countries throughout much of the developing world (Pauly and others 2006), where the figures are much higher because of the general lack of social insurance, a private insurance market, or employer-based health coverage. Given the lower income levels in these countries and the high proportion of medical expenditures paid out of pocket, payments that are small by U.S. standards likely will have large effects on behaviors in less developed countries. A further reason for patient-targeted performance-based incentive approaches is that prevention and treatment of many of the diseases that afflict large numbers of patients in developing countries such as HIV/AIDS, malaria, and tuberculosis (TB) require some component of change in the behavior of patients (as well as providers) to reduce the high rate of disease.

However, applying these concepts to developing countries involves additional challenges. One is that the public sector plays a larger role in service delivery, and an incentive-based approach would need to be integrated into an often-dysfunctional system of public provision. Information and communication infrastructures are less well developed, making identification and longitudinal patient follow-up more challenging. Logistical challenges to access and differing cultural views on health and western medical intervention may affect the population's ability and willingness to use health services in countries like the United States.

Here we focus on the applicability to developing countries of evidence from the United States on the utility of demand-side performance incentives in modifying patient health behavior. We discuss several considerations in designing patient-oriented pay-for-performance programs that may be important for developing countries.

Direct Evidence

Tests of performance-based financial rewards within the United States have shown the greatest effectiveness for changing short-term health behaviors. Numerous randomized controlled trials of incentive-based interventions have successfully increased the rate of follow-up visits in contexts ranging from abnormal pap smears (Marcus and others 1998) to postpartum visits by adolescents (Stevens-Simon, O'Connor, and Bassford 1994) and to rates at which patients with HIV return to learn the results of their purified protein derivative (PPD) tests (Chaisson and others 1996). In another example, the rate at which intravenous drug users received all three doses of hepatitis B vaccine was significantly higher among subjects receiving monetary incentives ($20 per month) than among those receiving outreach alone (69 and 23 percent, respectively, $p < 0 > 0.0001$; Seal and others 2002). Several studies show higher rates of tuberculin skin (PPD) test reading and completion of treatment among patients with tuberculosis. A randomized trial of 1,004 active or recent drug users found the rate of return for PPD test reading was 93 percent for those receiving $10 cash, 85 percent for those offered $5, 34 percent for those receiving motivational education, and 33 percent for those in the control group (Malotte, Rhodes, and Mais 1998). A monetary incentive of $5 increased the rate of reporting for an initial TB evaluation appointment among homeless people with positive tuberculin skin tests to 84 percent from the 53 percent among subjects in usual care ($p < 0.001$) and the 75 percent among those assigned to a peer health adviser (Pilote and others 1996). Forty-four percent (nineteen of forty-three) completed six months of isionazid therapy to 26 percent (ten of thirty-eight) in the usual care group ($p = 0.11$). The median number of months completed was five in the monetary incentive group, but only two in the peer health adviser group ($p = 0.005$) or the usual care group ($p = 0.04$; Tulsky and others 2000). These examples strongly suggest that this approach could be applied in developing countries, with probable large effects.

Performance-based financial incentives have been tested most extensively in substance abuse and have been successful in reducing rates of highly addictive behaviors such as alcohol, tobacco, and cocaine use (Higgins 1999; Higgins and Silverman 1999). Despite clear evidence from this literature (referred to as *contingency management*) that performance incentives have led to higher rates of retention in programs and abstinence (Higgins 1999), it is less clear that this approach is directly applicable to developing countries because these studies have been conducted in tightly controlled settings, such as drug treatment programs with frequent monitoring of subjects. One study, for example, randomized forty cocaine-using adults to either behavioral treatment or behavioral treatment plus vouchers exchangeable for retail items if urine samples were negative for cocaine during weeks one to twelve of the study (Higgins and others 1994). The groups were treated identically from weeks thirteen to twenty-four. Urine samples were collected three times a week, and subjects were eligible for progressively larger incentives the longer they stayed abstinent. The total potential value of the incentives was $997.50. Seventy-five percent of the incentive group completed treatment, compared with only 40 percent of the control group ($p = 0.03$). The incentive group demonstrated longer continuous abstinence both when receiving incentives and when not receiving them ($p < 0.05$) and did not relapse at greater rates once the incentives were discontinued.

The contingency management literature is characterized by similar studies. The effectiveness of incentives is clear, but frequent drug-level monitoring makes the approach difficult to export to less monitored settings. The literature clearly shows that the magnitude of the effect increases with the size of the incentive (Stitzer and Bigelow 1983, 1984; Higgins, Bickel, and Hughes 1994) and that delays in payment reduce the efficacy of incentives (Roll, Reilly, and Johanson 2000). Applying these approaches to less highly controlled settings has not been well tested, however (Petry and Simcic 2002). Contingency management approaches can be effective, but the need for frequent monitoring makes it seem less likely that this literature is directly applicable to the context of behavioral change for diseases in less developed countries.

The literature on performance incentives and smoking cessation, which has some potential applicability to less developed countries, is also extensive. The most applicable studies on smoking cessation have been randomized trials of narrowly targeted populations. One of pregnant and postpartum women offered a $50 voucher each month for saliva-cotinine-confirmed cessation by both the incentive group and their social supporters (Donatelle and others 2000). The incentive group had significantly higher quit rates during pregnancy than the control group

(32 and 9 percent, respectively, p < 0.0001). Eighty-seven percent had household incomes of less than $20,000. In a population of patients at a U.S. Department of Veterans Affairs medical center, financial incentives worth $200 increased cessation rates in the incentive group to 16.3 percent, compared with 4.6 percent in the control group (p < 0.001; Volpp and others 2006). The data from community settings are less useful because these studies have generally consisted of contests in which smokers were eligible to win prizes in a low-value lottery, often $1 or less. A review of seventeen tobacco studies noted that mean quit rates averaged 34 percent at one-month follow-up and about 23 percent at one-year follow-up (Bains, Pickett, and Hoey 1998). Such programs generally attract only 1 to 2 percent of the population, however, and because quit rates are generally measured conditional on enrollment in the program, the high rates likely reflect the highly skewed sample. In addition, quit rates have tended to be based on self-reports, without biochemical confirmation and with no control group for comparison (Fiore and others 2000).

Reviews have suggested that patient-targeted trials have generally been successful. A review from 1997 concluded that ten of eleven studies reviewed demonstrated that financial incentives promoted compliance better than any other tested alternative, which is particularly striking because all but one of the interventions provided incentives worth less than $50 (Giuffrida and Torgerson 1997). Most of these studies were geared toward keeping appointments and increasing immunization rates, but three successfully addressed health outcomes of blood pressure control, cocaine dependency, and obesity. A more recent review (Kane and others 2004) also highlights several areas in which further research is needed: the size of incentive needed to yield a major sustained effect, sustainability (because only four of forty-seven studies reviewed checked for long-term results and all of the measures that had improved significantly in the short term had returned to their original levels), and cost-effectiveness. Because only a small minority (seven of the forty-seven) included the necessary calculations, little is known about the cost-effectiveness of performance incentives (Kane and others 2004). Many of the ineffective interventions offered incentives worth less than $10 (Curry, Wagner, and Grothaus 1991). These reviews highlight both the strengths and limitations of this field: there is strong evidence for much broader implementation of interventions targeted at modifying short-term behaviors. More study is needed, however, on the effectiveness of different approaches in modifying longer-term behaviors, the responsiveness of behaviors to different incentives, and the cost effectiveness of different approaches.

One of the key empirical questions that require further investigation is whether behaviors will revert to baseline once payment stops. Two studies suggest that this could be a challenge. A small trial of fifty-five HIV patients found significant increases in adherence to antiretroviral medication (70 to 88 percent at week one) in the patients randomized to receive $2 per dose taken within two hours of the prescribed time. However, these improvements were not sustained when payment stopped after the fourth week (Rigsby and others 2000). When incentives were discontinued in a trial of smoking cessation, the difference at seventy-five days of 16.3 to 4.6 percent ($p < 0.0001$) narrowed to 6.5 to 4.6 percent at six months ($p = 0.57$; Volpp and others 2006). Incentives may provide extrinsic motivation during the intervention, but intrinsic motivation may not sustain the desired behavior (Curry, Wagner, and Grothaus 1991). The important question remains: how best to design performance-based approaches that achieve sustained behavioral change or that target behaviors where only short-term change is required.

Indirect Evidence

Non-performance-based financial incentives are both common and prima facie evidence that incentive-based approaches are important drivers of health behavior. Most of these incentives are manipulations of price rather than explicit rewards or penalties for specific behaviors, but we can also draw inferences in thinking about ways to modify health behavior in less developed countries.

Increases in excise taxes on tobacco products arguably have been the most successful approach to increasing the rate of tobacco cessation and discouraging people from beginning to smoke. A 10 percent increase in price results in about a 4 percent decrease in overall cigarette consumption (Chaloupka and Warner 2000). Higher prices for cigarettes make smokers less likely to smoke, which, though it now seems self-evident, had at one time been considered an unlikely presumption because of how highly addictive nicotine is (Grossman and others 1993; Chaloupka and Grossman 1996). It is also clear that full insurance coverage for tobacco cessation services increases both the use of services and the quit rates (Curry and others 1998). These studies show that smokers respond as rationally to differences in price as consumers of other goods and services. This suggests that incentive-based approaches can be effective when there is an addictive component and when there is not.

The most common use of incentives within U.S. health care settings has been financial and negative: incentives requiring patients to pay more across the board. These, such as copayments for medications, are common in employer-sponsored health insurance to reduce the use of services. Such untargeted incentives are used to discourage patients and physicians from relying on expensive drugs and ideally would only reduce the rate of inappropriate use of services. An extensive literature, however, documents less than ideal effects: significant reductions in the use of prescription drugs in response to relatively small increases in copayments, including for conditions such as hypertension for which daily medication is important (Leibowitz, Manning, and Newhouse 1985; Soumerai and others 1993; Joyce and others 2002; Steinman, Sands, and Covinsky 2001). This can contribute to worse health outcomes (Tamblyn and others 2001; Lurie and others 1984), particularly among low-income patients and those in poor health. The literature also shows reductions in the use of services, which seem to have little effect on health for populations that are neither poor nor at elevated risk (Newhouse 1996).

Less is known about the effects of targeted lowering of copayments as a tool to increase the use of beneficial or cost-effective services. This could be achieved by providing rewards that effectively lower the price of services, which could improve health cost-effectively (Coffield and others 2001). Such an approach is a form of benign moral hazard, in which enhanced coverage of services leads to higher use rates, but the higher rates are desired because the service is cost-effective in achieving better outcomes (Pauly and Held 1990). For example, full insurance coverage is associated with higher use rates of smoking cessation programs (2.4 percent with reduced coverage, 10 percent with full coverage) and higher quit rates (0.7 percent a year with reduced insurance coverage, 2.8 percent with full coverage; Curry and others 1998). The higher quit rates achieved with full coverage cost about $0.22 to $0.34 per enrollee per month. Although the cost savings from higher cessation rates might exceed the price to subsidize coverage of cessation, the focus should be on the fact that subsidization or rewards for such services are plausibly more cost-effective than many other commonly covered services.

Considerations

We draw on the U.S. experience to discuss several important issues related to designing and implementing incentive programs that need to be considered carefully in the context of less developed countries.

Priorities

Incentive programs should be considered based on public health consequences of the behavior, financial consequences of the behavior, the degree to which the behavior can be modified cost-effectively, and the duration of payments.

In the context of motivating adherence to treatment regimens, incentives are particularly compelling for diseases that pose significant health risks to a larger population. Tuberculosis is a clear example. Failure to adhere to therapy leads to prolonged infectivity through casual contact, generates transmissible drug-resistant pathogens, and dramatically increases the associated health costs. HIV transmission is analogous to TB transmission in some respects (Bangsberg, Mundy, and Tulsky 2001). Not adhering to therapy may also increase infectivity of both sensitive and drug-resistant viruses.

The financial consequences of detrimental health-related behaviors can take two forms: medical expenditures and workplace absenteeism and productivity. The Centers for Disease Control and Prevention has estimated that the economic costs of smoking in the United States total $3,391 per smoker per year and that more than half of this is lost productivity (CDC 2002). These figures were computed using data on changes in life expectancy and lifetime earnings, so they do not include the value of lost work time from smoking-related disability, absenteeism, and smoking breaks. Such savings are likely dwarfed in relative terms by the economic costs of HIV, malaria, and other common diseases in less developed countries that have an even higher disease burden than tobacco addiction.

The potential applicability of incentives to lowering the rates of unhealthy behaviors is relevant only if these behaviors can be modified cost-effectively. The incentives themselves can be cost-effective if used to modify health-related behaviors that frequently lead to expensive complications. The existing literature suggests that a wide range of behaviors can be modified with relatively inexpensive incentives (Giuffrida and Torgerson 1997). Smoking is an example of a disease that leads to expensive complications but for which cost-effective interventions are available but underused. Each year in the United States, $75 billion in medical services and an estimated $92 billion in lost productivity are attributable to smoking (CDC 2005). A wide range of cessation interventions have been found to have cost-effectiveness ratios below $20,000 per life-year saved, a much more favorable ratio than many health care services typically covered by health insurance and well below the commonly used coverage threshold of $50,000 to $100,000 per quality-adjusted life-year (Chernew, Hirth, and Cutler 2003). Blood pressure control has been shown to be highly cost-effective in reducing cardiovascular risk (Field and others 1995; Maynard 1992; Tsevat and others 1991), primarily because the multiple downstream effects of uncontrolled hypertension lead to large economic and social costs (Pardell and others 2000; McMurray 1999). The cost per life-year gained from treating hypertension may be as low as about $800, one of the lowest cost-effectiveness ratios observed for any medical treatment (Johannesson and others 1993).

The higher risk of adverse health outcomes in populations with higher levels of disease acuity suggests that incentive interventions should focus on modifying behavior in high-risk patients, such as encouraging the use of bed nets in endemic malaria areas or condoms among the sexually active in Sub-Saharan Africa. Whether this is true depends on the degree of behavioral change in response to interventions in these populations compared to lower-risk populations. Ideally, efforts of both lower and higher intensity would be directed at different populations, because different types of interventions could complement one another and the intensity of the intervention will depend on the resources available. What is not known is whether incentives can be systematically used to enhance the use of such services and whether the incentives themselves will be cost-effective.

Empirical evidence in favor of programs with time-limited interventions is much stronger than that for programs with longer-term interventions. Feasibility is greatest with those that target increasing vaccinations for influenza, hepatitis B, or other infectious diseases, which generally require only one to three points of contact. Incentive-based approaches to increasing the completion of tuberculosis treatment have also been effective, because, although they require months, most patients are cured. Incentives to improve health-related behavior for chronic diseases, such as HIV or hypertension, are less favorable in this regard.

Approaches

Different approaches can be taken to encourage healthy behaviors. One is to use differential risk rating, tying insurance premiums to personal health behavior. This is an option only in systems with a high proportion of people with private health insurance, however. Another is to offer price discounts for highly cost-effective services to encourage their use. The third is to offer rewards that encourage specific behaviors. It seems possible that unbundling rewards may have larger effects than lowering insurance premiums because of endowment effects and status quo bias. Ideally these approaches would be tested head to head. Given the low incomes in less developed countries, however, it seems likely that both would be highly effective.

Nature of Incentive

Noncash incentives are often used because of concerns that giving money to those with substance abuse problems is an unseemly risk. Some evidence, however, indicates that an equivalent amount of cash might be more effective. A randomized trial of 1,078 active drug users found that the rate of return for PPD skin test reading was 95 percent for those receiving $10 cash, 86 percent for those receiving grocery store coupons, 83 percent for those receiving either bus tokens or fast-food coupons, 47 percent for those receiving an educational session, and 49 percent for those receiving simply encouragement. Differences between the cash incentive and the grocery store coupon were significant (chi-square 9.5, $p = 0.002$) as were those between cash and the bus pass or food coupon (chi-square 15.4, $p < 0.0001$; Malotte, Hollingshead, and Rhodes 1999). In a study that examined attendance at an AIDS prevention program, a shift from monetary payments to vouchers for food or gifts led to a substantial decline in attendance (Dern and others 1994). Cash payments have the added benefit of letting the subject decide how to spend the money, and, as in the context of Christmas presents (Waldfogel 1993), subjects may value gifts at substantially less than the amount spent on them, making noncash incentive payments considerably less efficient. A further advantage to cash is that considerable staff time is needed if in-kind gifts are provided in lieu of cash.

Administration

Turnover in private insurance markets and among employers is one reason for underinvestment in prevention within the United States. Insurers and employers are reluctant to invest in prevention if the savings in future medical expenditures accrue to someone else. Such programs will likely be broadly adopted only if doing so makes financial sense for employers and insurers. The potential in less developed countries for employers to contribute to health promotion efforts may be greater because of the clear implications of many common diseases such as malaria and HIV for absenteeism and productivity for firms.

Incentive programs are applied most favorably in cases with high short-term payoffs (better asthma management), a compelling public health rationale because of contagious disease (multidrug-resistant TB), or within health systems or insurers with low turnover (such as Medicare). Employers with low turnover could consider adopting such policies on either an individual or a group basis. When there are enough externalities either in terms of public health (multidrug-resistant TB) or financial consequences (smoking), if turnover between firms creates a free-rider problem, consideration could be given to mandating coverage across all insurers or employers within a region.

Sustainability

For sustained change in health behaviors, an important decision is whether payments need to be continued indefinitely or whether incentives can be dropped.

Motivational theory and previous empirical work suggest that incentives may bring people into treatment but do not necessarily lead to higher success rates (Curry, Wagner, and Grothaus 1991). It is generally thought that sustained behavioral change is unlikely without some intrinsic motivation.

Context

Incentive approaches in the United States for diseases such as tuberculosis, which kills almost 3 million people a year, mostly in low-income countries, are directly applicable to less developed countries. Treatment completion rates in general are not high, however. Even within the United States, about 44 percent of TB patients do not complete therapy (CDC, American Thoracic Society, and Infectious Diseases Society of America 2005). This can result in prolonged infectiousness, relapse, drug resistance, and death. Other leading killers in less developed countries, such as HIV and malaria, may require new approaches. Using incentives for ongoing behavior to reduce risks or increase compliance with HIV treatment regimens is an important area for further research.

Equity-Fairness

Incentives are most efficient if targeted at those whose behavior needs to change. This targeting can raise equity and fairness issues if those who are already practicing desired behavior feel that incentives penalize them for good behavior. One approach to consider is to give members of a given community points to lose for unhealthy behavior. An argument can also be made, from the standpoints of both cost and personal risk, that everyone in a given collective (HIV-negative individuals) potentially benefits when higher-risk individuals (HIV-positive individuals who do not adhere to safe practices) change their behavior.

Managing Data

Systems need to be set up to identify the appropriate participants, deliver the promised incentives, account for the flow of dollars, and measure the effects on use and outcomes. Mechanisms are needed to verify that the behaviors in question did, in fact, change and to ensure that the dollars flow in a timely manner to those who modify the desired behavior. Less will be demanded of the data infrastructure in setting up such programs for one-time behaviors such as influenza vaccines, in which compliance and payment can be measured at the point of service. Verifying behavioral change becomes increasingly difficult with the degree to which the behavior is not observed. Attendance for vaccines or postpartum visits is easy to measure, but verification of the use of mosquito netting is harder to ascertain other than through random audits. How best to measure adherence given differences in local customs and cultures needs to be considered carefully.

Rigorous Evaluation

It is essential that any new efforts be tested through rigorous quasi-experimental or experimental designs so that the effectiveness and cost-effectiveness of these early efforts can be measured. It is of central importance to the further improvement of existing approaches to build into the design of pay-for-performance programs rigorous evaluation of their impact as well as ongoing qualitative assessments so that potential problems can be identified and proactively addressed.

Conclusions

There are several conclusions to draw. Patient-targeted pay for performance is effective in changing short-term behavior. Whether this approach is cost-effective is still unclear, but several comparative studies indicate that it is significantly more so than other commonly used approaches, such as education or peer support.

This suggests an initial focus on increasing the use of services that are known to be beneficial and cost-effective but that require few points of contact. Examples include childhood immunizations, PPD test reading, and distribution of malaria nets. Incentives to improve adherence to a time-limited course of treatment for diseases such as tuberculosis in which lack of treatment poses a clear risk to the health of others would be another logical target. Incentives to increase the use of medications for chronic diseases such as HIV would also be important, but probably would entail indefinite price reductions to ensure adherence.

The high proportion of medical expenditures that are paid out of pocket in developing countries is evidence enough that cost of services is a major issue of access. Patient-targeted performance incentives would help to reduce these barriers and could complement provider-targeted incentives. Extremely high expenditures and misaligned incentives in the United States have generally not produced high rates of healthy behavior, and this is a lesson for developing countries. Consideration should be given to building private-public partnerships in part because employers would benefit greatly from reducing absenteeism as a result of the many diseases endemic within much of the population.

References

American Heart Association. 2002. *Heart and Stroke Statistical Update.* Dallas. (www.american heart.org/downloadable/heart/HS_State_02.pdf [October 2008].)

Amery, Antoon, and others. 1985. "Mortality and Morbidity Results from the European Working Party on High Blood Pressure in the Elderly Trial." *Lancet* 1 (8442):1349–54.

Bains, Namrata, William Pickett, and John Hoey. 1998. "The Use and Impact of Incentives in Population-Based Smoking Cessation Programs: A Review." *American Journal of Health Promotion* 12 (5): 307–20.

Bangsberg, David R., Linda M. Mundy, and Jacqueline P. Tulsky. 2001. "Expanding Directly Observed Therapy: Tuberculosis to Human Immunodeficiency Virus." *American Journal of Medicine* 110 (8): 664–66.

Bartlett, Joan, Leonard Miller, Dorothy Rice, and Wendy Max. 1994. "Medical Care Expenditures Attributable to Cigarette Smoking: United States, 1993." *Morbidity and Mortality Weekly Report* 43 (26): 469–72.

CDC (Centers for Disease Control and Prevention). 2002. "Annual Smoking-Attributable Mortality, Years of Potential Life Lost, and Economic Costs: United States, 1995–1999." *Morbidity and Mortality Weekly Report* 51 (14): 300–03.

———. 2005. "Annual Smoking-Attributable Mortality, Years of Potential Life Lost, and Productivity Losses: United States, 1997–2001." *Morbidity and Mortality Weekly Report* 54 (25): 625–28.

CDC, American Thoracic Society, and Infectious Diseases Society of America. 2005. "Controlling Tuberculosis in the United States." *American Journal of Respiratory Critical Care Medicine* 172 (9): 1169–227.

Chaisson, R. E., J. C. Keruly, S. McAvinue, J. E. Gallant, and R. D. Moore. 1996. "Effects of an Incentive and Education Program on Return Rates for PPD Test Treating in Patients with HIV Infection." *Journal of Acquired Immune Deficiency Syndromes and Human Retrovirology* 11: 455–59.

Chaloupka, Frank J., and Michael Grossman. 1996. "Price, Tobacco Control Policies, and Youth Smoking." NBER Working Paper 5740. Cambridge, Mass.: National Bureau of Economic Research.

Chaloupka, Frank J., and K. E. Warner. 2000. "The Economics of Smoking." In *The Handbook of Health Economics,* edited by J. P. Newhouse and A. J. Culyer. New York: Elsevier.

Chernew, Michael E., Richard A. Hirth, and David M. Cutler. 2003. "Increased Spending on Health Care: How Much Can the United States Afford?" *Health Affairs* 22 (4): 15–25.

Coffield, A. B., M. V. Maciosek, J. M. McGinnis, and others. 2001. "Priorities among Recommended Clinical Preventive Services." *American Journal of Preventive Medicine* 21 (1): 1–9.

Curry, S. J., L. C. Grothaus, T. McAfee, and others. 1998. "Use and Cost-Effectiveness of Smoking-Cessation Services under Four Insurance Plans in a Health Maintenance Organization." *New England Journal of Medicine* 339 (10): 673–79.

Curry, Susan J., Edward H. Wagner, and Louis C. Grothaus. 1991. "Evaluation of Intrinsic and Extrinsic Motivation Interventions with a Self-Help Smoking Cessation Program." *Journal of Consulting and Clinical Psychology* 59 (2): 318–24.

Dern, S., R. Stephens, W. R. Davis, T. E. Feucht, and S. Tortu. 1994. "The Impact of Providing Incentives for Attendance at AIDS Prevention Sessions." *Public Health Reports* 109 (4): 548–54.

DiMatteo, M. R. 2004. "Variations in Patients' Adherence to Medical Recommendations: A Quantitative Review of 50 Years of Research." *Medical Care* 42 (3): 200–09.

Donatelle, Rebecca J., and others. 2000. "Randomised Controlled Trial Using Social Support and Financial Incentives for High Risk Pregnant Smokers: Significant Other Supporter (SOS) Program." *International Journal of Tobacco Control—Journal of the British Medical Association* 9 (III): 67–71.

Eisen, S. A., D. K. Miller, R. S. Woodward, E. Spitznagel, and T. R. Przybeck. 1990. "The Effect of Prescribed Daily Dose Frequency on Patient Medication Compliance." *Archives of Internal Medicine* 150 (9): 1881–84.

Field, K., M. Thorogood, C. Silagy, C. Normand, C. O'Neill, and J. Muir. 1995. "Strategies for Reducing Coronary Risk Factors in Primary Care: Which Is Most Cost-Effective?" *British Medical Journal* 310 (6987): 1109–12.

Fiore, M. C., W. C. Bailey, S. J. Cohen, and others. 2000. *Treating Tobacco Use and Dependence: Clinical Practice Guideline.* Rockville, Md.: U.S. Department of Health and Human Services, Public Health Service.

Giuffrida, Antonio, and David J. Torgerson. 1997. "Should We Pay the Patient? Review of Financial Incentives to Enhance Patient Compliance." *British Medical Journal* 315 (7110): 703–07.

Grossman, Michael, J. L. Sindelar, J. Mullahy, and R. Anderson. 1993. "Policy Watch: Alcohol and Cigarette Taxes." *Journal of Economic Perspectives* 7 (4): 211–22.

Higgins, S. T. 1999. "Applying Behavioral Economics to the Challenge of Reducing Cocaine Abuse." In *The Economic Analysis of Substance Use and Abuse,* edited by Frank Chaloupa and others. Cambridge, Mass.: National Bureau of Economic Research.

Higgins, Stephen T., W. K. Bickel, and J. R. Hughes. 1994. "Influence of an Alternative Reinforcer on Human Cocaine Self-Administration." *Life Science* 55 (3): 179–87.

Higgins, Stephen T., A. J. Budney, W. K. Bickel, F. E. Foerg, R. Donham, and G. Badger. 1994. "Incentives Improve Outcomes in Outpatient Behavioral Treatment of Cocaine Dependence." *Archives of General Psychiatry* 51 (7): 568–76.

Higgins, Stephen T., and Kenneth Silverman, eds. 1999. *Motivating Behavior Change among Illicit Drug Abusers: Research on Contingency Management Interventions.* Washington: American Psychological Association.

Hughes, John R. 2003. "Motivating and Helping Smokers to Stop Smoking." *Journal of General Internal Medicine* 18 (12): 1053–57.

Johannesson, M., B. Dahlof, L. H. Lindholm, and others. 1993. "The Cost-Effectiveness of Treating Hypertension in Elderly People: An Analysis of the Swedish Trial in Old Patients with Hypertension (STOP Hypertension)." *Journal of Internal Medicine* 234 (3): 317–23.

Joyce, Geoffrey F., J. J. Escarce, M. D. Solomon, and D. P. Goldman. 2002. "Employer Drug Benefit Plans and Spending on Prescription Drugs." *Journal of the American Medical Association* 288 (14): 1733–39.

Kane, Robert L., P. E. Johnson, R. J. Town, and M. Butler. 2004. "A Structured Review of the Effect of Economic Incentives on Consumers' Preventive Behavior." *American Journal of Preventive Medicine* 27 (4): 327–52.

Klag, Michael J., P. K. Whelton, B. L. Randall, and others. 1996. "Blood Pressure and End-Stage Renal Disease in Men." *New England Journal of Medicine* 334 (1): 13–18.

Leibowitz, Arleen, Willard G. Manning, and Joseph P. Newhouse. 1985. "The Demand for Prescription Drugs as a Function of Cost-Sharing." *Social Science Medicine* 21 (10): 1063–69.

Lurie, Nicole, N. B. Ward, M. F. Shapiro, and R. H. Brook. 1984. "Termination from Medi-Cal: Does It Affect Health?" *New England Journal of Medicine* 311 (7): 480–84.

Malotte, C. Kevin, J. R. Hollingshead, and F. Rhodes. 1999. "Monetary Versus Nonmonetary Incentives for TB Skin Test Reading among Drug Users." *American Journal of Preventive Medicine* 16 (3): 182–88.

Malotte, C. Kevin, F. Rhodes, and K. E. Mais. 1998. "Tuberculosis Screening and Compliance with Return for Skin Test Reading among Active Drug Users." *American Journal of Public Health* 88 (5): 792–96.

Marcus, Alfred, C. P. Kaplan, L. A. Crane, J. S. Berek, G. Bernstein, and J. E. Gunning. 1998. "Reducing Loss to Follow-up among Women with Abnormal Pap Smears: Results from a Randomized Trial Testing an Intensive Follow-up Protocol and Economic Incentives." *Medical Care* 36 (3): 397.

Maynard, Alan. 1992. "The Economics of Hypertension Control: Some Basic Issues." *Journal of Human Hypertension* 6 (6): 417–20.

McDonald, Heather P., Amit X. Garg, and R. Brian Haynes. 2002. "Interventions to Enhance Patient Adherence to Medication Prescriptions: Scientific Review." *Journal of the American Medical Association* 288 (22): 2868–79.

McMurray, J. 1999. "The Health Economics of the Treatment of Hyperlipidemia and Hypertension." *American Journal of Hypertension* 12 (10, supplement): S99–104.

Mokdad, Ali H., J. S. Marks, D. F. Stroup, and J. L. Gerberding. 2004. "Actual Causes of Death in the United States, 2000." *Journal of the American Medical Association* 291 (10): 1238–45.

Monane, M., R. L. Bohn, J. H. Gurwitz, R. J. Glynn, R. Levin, and J. Avorn. 1996. "Compliance with Antihypertensive Therapy among Elderly Medicaid Enrollees: The Roles of Age, Gender, and Race." *American Journal of Public Health* 86 (12): 1805–08.

Nelson, E. C., W. B. Stason, R. R. Neutra, and H. S. Solomon. 1980. "Identification of the Noncompliant Hypertensive Patient." *Preventive Medicine* 9 (4): 504–17.

Newhouse, Joseph P. 1996. *Free for All? Lessons from the Rand Health Insurance Experiment.* Harvard University Press.

Pardell, Helios, R. Tresserras, P. Armario, and D. R. Hernandez. 2000. "Pharmacoeconomic Considerations in the Management of Hypertension." *Drugs* 59 (supplement 2): 13–20.

Pauly, Mark V., and Philip J. Held. 1990. "Benign Moral Hazard and the Cost-Effectiveness Analysis of Insurance Coverage." *Journal of Health Economics* 9 (4): 447–61.

Pauly, Mark V., P. Zweifel, R. M. Scheffler, A. S. Preker, and M. Bassett. 2006. "Private Health Insurance in Developing Countries." *Health Affairs* 25 (2): 369–79.

Petry, Nancy M., and Francis Simcic. 2002. "Recent Advances in the Dissemination of Contingency Management Techniques: Clinical and Research Perspectives." *Journal of Substance Abuse Treatment* 23 (2): 81–86.

Pilote, L., J. P. Tulsky, A. R. Zolopa, J. A. Hahn, G. F. Schecter, and A. R. Moss. 1996. "Tuberculosis Prophylaxis in the Homeless: A Trial to Improve Adherence to Referral." *Archives of Internal Medicine* 156 (2): 161–65.

Rigsby, Michael O., M. I. Rosen, J. E. Beauvais, J. A. Cramer, P. M. Rainey, S. S. O'Malley, K. D. Dieckhaus, and B. J. Rounsaville. 2000. "Cue-Dose Training with Monetary Reinforcement." *Journal of General Internal Medicine* 15 (12): 841–47.

Roll, J. M., M. P. Reilly, and C.-E. Johanson. 2000. "The Influence of Exchange Delays on Cigarette versus Money Choice: A Laboratory Analog of Voucher-Based Reinforcement Therapy." *Experimental and Clinical Psychopharmacology* 8 (3): 366–70.

Seal, Karen H., Alex H. Kral, Jennifer Lorvick, Alex McNees, Lauren Gee, and Brian R. Edlin. 2002. "A Randomized Controlled Trial of Monetary Incentives vs. Outreach to Enhance Adherence to the Hepatitis B Vaccine Series among Injection Drug Users." *Drug and Alcohol Dependence* 71 (2): 127–31.

SHEP (Systolic Hypertension in the Elderly Program), Cooperative Research Group. 1991. "Prevention of Stroke by Antihypertensive Drug Treatment in Older Persons with Isolated Systolic Hypertension. Final Results of the Systolic Hypertension in the Elderly Program (SHEP)." *Journal of the American Medical Association* 265 (24): 3255–64.

Soumerai, S. B., D. Ross-Degnan, E. E. Fortess, and J. Abelson. 1993. "A Critical Analysis of Studies of State Drug Reimbursement Policies: Research in Need of Discipline." *Milbank Quarterly* 71 (2): 217–52.

Steinman, Michael A., Laura P. Sands, and Kenneth E. Covinsky. 2001. "Self-Restriction of Medications Due to Cost in Seniors without Prescription Coverage." *Journal of General Internal Medicine* 16 (12): 793–99.

Stevens-Simon, C., Patrick O'Connor, and Karen Bassford. 1994. "Incentives Enhance Postpartum Compliance among Adolescent Prenatal Patients." *Journal of Adolescent Health* 15 (5): 396–99.

Stitzer, Maxine L., and G. E. Bigelow. 1983. "Contingent Payment for Carbon Monoxide Reduction: Effects of Pay Amount." *Behavior Therapy* 14 (2): 647–56.

———. 1984. "Contingent Reinforcement for Carbon Monoxide Reduction: Within-Subject Effects of Pay Amount." *Journal of Applied Behavior Analysis* 17 (4): 477–83.

Tamblyn, Robyn, R. Laprise, J. A. Hanley, and others. 2001. "Adverse Events Associated with Prescription Drug Cost-Sharing among Poor and Elderly Persons." *Journal of the American Medical Association* 285 (4): 421–29.

Tsevat, J., M. C. Weinstein, L. W. Williams, A. N. Tosteson, and L. Goldman. 1991. "Expected Gains in Life Expectancy from Various Coronary Heart Disease Risk Factor Modifications." *Circulation* 83 (4): 1194–201.

Tulsky, Jacqueline P., L. P. Pilote, J. A. Hahn, A. J. Zolopa, M. Burke, M. Chesney, and A. R. Moss. 2000. "Adherence to Isoniazid Prophylaxis in the Homeless: A Randomized Controlled Trial." *Archives of Internal Medicine* 160 (5): 697–702.

Volpp, Kevin G., A. Gurmankin, J. Berlin, and others. 2006. "A Randomized Controlled Trial of Financial Incentives for Smoking Cessation." *Cancer, Epidemiology, Biomarkers, and Prevention* 15 (1): 12–18.

Waldfogel, Joel. 1993. "The Deadweight Loss of Christmas." *American Economic Review* 83 (5): 1328–36.

8

Afghanistan: Paying NGOs for Performance in a Postconflict Setting

Egbert Sondorp, Natasha Palmer, Lesley Strong, and Abdul Wali

---

Highlights

Large-scale contracting of nongovernmental organizations can deliver essential services to the population, even in a postconflict setting with weak service delivery capacity.

Government stewardship of the health sector can be enhanced with services delivered by contracted nongovernmental organizations.

Results suggest that nongovernmental organizations that are paid based partly on results perform better than those that are paid for expenditures on inputs, although this evidence is far from conclusive.

In 2002 donors and the nascent Afghan Ministry of Public Health decided to contract nongovernmental organizations (NGOs) to provide access to a defined package of essential health services. The three major donors active in the health sector—the European Commission (EC), the U.S. Agency for International Development (USAID), and the World Bank—varied in their approaches to payment, technical assistance, and accountability, which presented a wonderful opportunity to compare the effectiveness of alternative approaches. The World Bank incorporated performance bonuses in addition to a reliable fixed payment and allowed recipients to use funds in ways they deemed to be most effective. Other donors reimbursed for documented expenditures on inputs, without an explicit performance-related financial incentive, and imposed rigidities on the use of funds. Each approach required NGOs to report and account differently for performance, and each donor provided access to different forms of technical assistance. This case, therefore, offers an opportunity to contrast the effectiveness of payment for performance with input-based payment in a postconflict setting and to explore implementation issues.

We describe the different contractual approaches and explore the limited evidence on their effectiveness. The available evidence suggests that those providers being paid with a pay-for-performance element in their contract perform better in some areas than NGO providers being paid with other mechanisms. The methods used to assess performance show some weaknesses, however, as do the measures of performance themselves, making it difficult to draw conclusions about the effectiveness of payment for performance in this complex picture. For example, location-specific factors such as security, geography, and baseline conditions at each facility may partly or fully explain observed differences in performance.

Background

Afghanistan has had some of the worst health statistics in the world for almost half a century. Even in the 1960s and 1970s, the health of Afghan women and children was far behind that of others in the region, and health services were largely absent in rural areas (Strong, Wali, and Sondorp 2005). This situation worsened as a result of years of conflict. The United Nations Children Fund's multiple indicator cluster surveys for 1997 and 2000 placed Afghanistan as having the fourth highest rates of child and infant mortality in the world. One child in four dies before he or she is five years old (Fleck 2004). The country's recent national survey of maternal mortality estimated maternal mortality at 1,600 per 100,000, on average, but the range varies between 400 and 6,500 per 100,000 across regions (Bartlett and others 2005), the second highest rate in the world. Inadequate human resources in the health sector present another extreme challenge: Afghanistan has only one doctor per 2,500 people and a severe shortage of trained midwives; only one in five nurses is female (Ministry of Public Health, Management Sciences for Health 2002).

Following the fall of the Taliban regime in 2001, donors began to review possible approaches to building up Afghanistan's barely functioning health system.

Table 8-1. *Contracts Awarded in Afghanistan, by Donors since 2003*

Donor	Number of grants or contracts	Number of provinces	Population	Coverage (percent)	Annual costs per capita (U.S. dollars)[a]
USAID	30	14	6,711,526	33	4.82[b]
European Commission	13	40	4,031,000	20	5.22
World Bank MoPH-SM	8	8	3,585,000	18	3.80
World Bank-PPA	1	3	1,105,247	5	4.82
Asian Development Bank	3	3	294,500	1	4.83
Totals	55	34	15,727,273	77	4.68

Source: Authors.
a. Bid prices.
b. USAID bid excludes drug costs.

The first joint donor review mission in 2002 highlighted the possibility of contracting NGOs to provide health services under the stewardship of the Ministry of Public Health. This would fit both the policy intention to create a lean government and the reality on the ground, where the majority of health services (estimated at 80 percent) were being provided by a number of well-established NGOs. The notion of using output-based incentives was also introduced, and the proposed contracts were referred to as performance-based partnership agreements. NGOs would compete to win contracts to provide a basic package of health services to people living in a geographically defined area. The Ministry of Public Health officially endorsed the approach, and the first contracts and grants were signed in 2003. All major donors in the health sector subscribed to this approach, but from the start some differences among donors were visible, primarily motivated by institutional arrangements internal to each agency (Strong, Wali, and Sondorp 2006a).

In collaboration with the Ministry of Public Health, between 2003 and 2005, the European Commission, the World Bank, and USAID entered into contracts with NGOs worth more than $155 million to provide the basic package of health services in regions covering 77 percent of the population. Between 2003 and late 2005, fifty-five contracts were awarded in a series of bidding rounds. Some details on these contracts are given in table 8-1. The Asian Development Bank (ADB) funded several contracts, also shown, but these were small in comparison to those of the other donors, and there are no plans to finance more. We do not include discussion of ADB contracts because they are of marginal importance in future plans for contracts in Afghanistan.

Donor Approaches

Although the basic package of health services and contracts with NGOs for its delivery are common to all approaches, the nature of the contract used to govern the relationship differs among the donors. This variation is reflected in the use of quite different terminology, ranging from the European Commission calling them grants to the World Bank calling them performance-based partnership agreements. We refer to them generally as contracts (see table 8-2 for more detail on the various mechanisms).

The World Bank

World Bank funds service delivery through two types of contracts: those with NGOs to provide the basic package of health services to an entire province and those with the Ministry of Public Health to deliver services in three provinces through the so-called strengthening mechanism (MoPH-SM). The World Bank is the only donor to incorporate performance-based incentives as defined in this volume. Performance-based partnership agreements offer the prospect of winning a bonus worth 10 percent (amounting to more than $800,000 in some cases) of the contract value as an incentive to reach or exceed specified targets. This is achievable in stages, with 1 percent of the contract value payable for at least a 10 percent increase from the baseline for specified indicators. The final 5 percent bonus is paid at the end of the contract. By 2007 interim performance bonuses had been awarded to three NGOs, and more NGOs are expected to receive the bonus. In addition, the Ministry of Public Health is expected to earn a bonus for performance in the three provinces where the contracts are funded through the strengthening mechanism.

These contracts allow relative flexibility in how funds are spent, but they are still subject to the National Salary Policy and the tight specifications of the basic package of health services, which details services, staffing patterns, and ratios of facility to population. World Bank managers emphasized that this type of contract decentralizes authority to field managers and encourages innovation, because providers are motivated to reach performance targets by the autonomy and associated flexibility to use funds effectively and efficiently as well as by the opportunity to earn performance bonuses. The World Bank approach does not provide formal technical assistance, but its monitoring missions do offer frequent feedback.

Table 8-2. *Summary of Features of Approaches in Afghanistan*

Features and time period	USAID	World Bank/Ministry of Public Health		European Commission
		NGOs	*Ministry of Public Health strengthening mechanism*	
Type 2002–05	Term used by donor: performance-based grant. Cost reimbursement against budget line items, with limited flexibility between items	Term used by donor: performance-based partnership agreement. Fixed lump-sum remuneration with 100 percent budget flexibility, with possibility of earning up to 10 percent of contract price in bonus	Term used by donor: performance-based partnership agreement. Set up as specific project within Ministry of Public Health, but will use regular government procedures; certain elements subcontracted to NGOs. Fixed lump-sum remuneration with 100 percent budget flexibility; possibility of earning up to 10 percent of contract price in bonus	Term used by donor: grant contract; cost reimbursed against line-item expenditure. NGOs required to contribute 20 percent of the overall budget (but mostly waived)
Plans for 2006 onward	To be called performance-based partnership grants; same budget and payment mechanisms	Same	Same	Cost reimbursement, but based on more detailed reporting of outputs

(continued)

Table 8-2. *Summary of Features of Approaches in Afghanistan (continued)*

Features and time period	World Bank/Ministry of Public Health			European Commission
	USAID	*NGOs*	*Ministry of Public Health strengthening mechanism*	
Geographic scope of coverage				
2002–05	Fourteen provinces; cluster-wide coverage: clusters of districts are recommended, but NGOs can propose their own clusters or even one district for funding. Other parts of the province may not be covered by a contract	Eight provinces; province-wide coverage: one basic package of health services provider in one province. They may work in partnership with other NGOs	Three provinces; province-wide coverage	Ten provinces; mix of cluster and province-wide approaches
Plans for 2006 onward	Thirteen provinces; three province-wide performance-based partnership grants; eighteen cluster-wide performance-based partnership grants (nine provinces): districts are predefined and cannot be altered	Province-wide coverage in eight provinces; the World Bank will expand coverage in several uncovered clusters in other provinces in early 2006	Province-wide coverage in three provinces; plans to expand the strengthening mechanism to four uncovered districts of Kabul	Mix of cluster and province-wide approaches in ten provinces; European Commission responsible for all of Ghor province
Duration				
2002–05	Twelve to thirty-six months	Twenty-six to thirty-six months	Twenty-four months	Twenty-one to thirty months
Plans for 2006 onward	Thirty months, with the possibility to extend for the same time period if performance is good for a total of five years	Eighteen-month extensions on existing contracts and twenty-four-month contracts for new providers	Eighteen-month extension	All areas will come up for tendering again during 2007

Performance-based elements

2002–05	Performance-based grant: payment can be withheld if deliverables outlined in the contract are not met, but there is no monetary bonus	Performance-based partnership agreement: monetary bonus of 10 percent of the contract value over the life of the project. 1 percent awarded every six months for increases of 10 percentage points above baseline (for a total of 5 percent over the project) plus an additional 5 percent at the end of the project for improvements of at least 50 percentage points. Provincial health officers will be eligible to receive a bonus if NGOs qualify for a bonus	Same as NGO: monetary bonus of 10 percent of the contract value over the life of the project. 1 percent awarded every six months for increases of 10 percentage points above baseline (for a total of 5 percent over the project) plus an additional 5 percent at the end of the project for improvements of at least 50 percentage points	No performance-based components to date
Plans for 2006 onward	Performance-based partnership grant; there is still no monetary bonus, but extension of projects for an additional 2.5 years (for a project total of five years) is contingent on performance in line with expectations		Same	Plans to instate "service contracts," where reimbursement of expenses is contingent on achievement of outputs. However, last-minute decision to revert back to "grant contracts"

(continued)

Table 8-2. *Summary of Features of Approaches in Afghanistan (continued)*

Features and time period	USAID	World Bank/Ministry of Public Health		European Commission
		NGOs	Ministry of Public Health strengthening mechanism	
Reporting, monitoring, and evaluation				
2002–05	Monthly review of deliverables through reports and spontaneous on-site monitoring and evaluation. The fully functional service delivery point quality improvement monitoring tool has been implemented in 65 percent of REACH facilities; baseline, midterm, and end of project household survey using Lot Quality Assurance Sampling methodology to measure outputs	Nationwide annual household surveys and facility-based inspections or interviews and semiannual facility inspections in all performance-based partnership agreements and province-wide projects conducted by third-party evaluator (Johns Hopkins University, IIHMR); submission of quarterly narrative and financial reports; ad hoc missions of World Bank and Ministry of Public Health	Same	Submission of annual reports to the European Commission and quarterly submission of technical narrative reports to the Ministry of Public Health as of late 2004
Plans for 2006 onward	Routine monitoring activities will remain more or less the same, although not at the same magnitude. Data from the final Household Health Surveys will be used as the baseline for new projects,	Johns Hopkins University–IIHMR contract has been extended to continue with the same scheme until 2008	Same	Semiannual reports to the Ministry of Public Health and the EC and external evaluation and quality assessment of the contracted basic package of health services projects

	and targets will be negotiated with NGOs. Evaluation will most likely be conducted by an external body			

Indicators

2002–05	USAID has set standard indicators, but the targets can be defined by the NGO and negotiated with the purchaser. Baseline figures are based on household surveys conducted by the NGOs in the first quarter of the grant	Nationally defined core and management indicators. Baseline figures will be extracted from a multiple indicator cluster survey conducted in 2003	Same	NGOs can define their own indicators and use a traditional logical framework. However, one of the priorities of the program is to start defining and measuring performance-based indicators related to the basic package of health services
Plans for 2006 onward	Indicators will be revised to include a mixture of previous USAID standard indicators and PPA indicators. Targets are still set by the NGO and negotiated with the purchaser	Indicators will be revised based on feasibility of data collection on current indicators	Same	Indicators will be based on national indicators, to be made province-specific

Source: Strong, Wali, and Sondorp (2006a).

The World Bank is the only donor that channels funds through the Afghan Ministry of Finance; the Ministry of Public Health is responsible for paying contractors. The Ministry of Public Health also carried out the procurement process, subject to approval by the World Bank. A Ministry of Public Health unit is responsible for collecting quarterly health data for ongoing monitoring. To complement this, independent monitoring and evaluation are contracted to a third party made up of Johns Hopkins University and the Indian Institute of Health Management Research.

USAID

USAID's Rural Expansion of Afghanistan's Community-based Healthcare (REACH) project has awarded contracts to NGOs to deliver the basic package of health services with the Management Sciences for Health as the implementing agency. REACH awards two types of contracts: those to NGOs to deliver services in single districts or clusters of districts and those to implementing partners and the Ministry of Public Health to deliver technical assistance. Unlike the World Bank, REACH permits multiple providers in a province. REACH has an explicit focus on capacity building, so attention has been paid to establishing new and improving the management systems of existing national NGOs.

Management Sciences for Health representatives in Afghanistan felt that in the first phase of funding NGOs were not prepared to operate successfully under pay for performance and wanted to see how well NGOs could function without incentives. Because they believed that introducing monetary incentives would create opportunities for fraud, they thought that efforts should focus on improving the technical capacity of NGOs to deliver the basic package of health services.

Under the REACH project, therefore, NGOs establish targets for improvement for a standardized set of indicators—a mix of input, process, and output indicators—developed by Management Sciences for Health. Performance is measured against these indicators, but there is no performance-based bonus. Payment can be withheld if deliverables (monthly reports) are not submitted or if monitoring visits reveal problems. Contracts can also be terminated for failure to perform. This has happened once.

Although Management Sciences for Health ran the procurement process in the initial round, the Ministry of Public Health was involved in all stages, including development of tender documents and evaluation of bids. Both central- and provincial-level representatives of the ministry were included in the evaluation. Although monitoring activities and grant management were responsibilities of Management Sciences for Health in the initial round of grants (between 2002 and mid-2006), USAID handed over these tasks to the Ministry of Public Health in the second round. Institutional procurement rules continue to prevent USAID from channeling funds through the government. The World Health Organization will manage payments for the second round of contracts.

EUROPEAN COMMISSION

The European Commission was the first donor to contract NGOs to deliver health services in early 2003, before the final version of the basic package of health services was approved. Contracts awarded to date do not contain any performance-based features, and the EC approach most closely resembles traditional grant funding. A competitive process was put in place to award contracts, but NGOs are reimbursed for expenditures on inputs. NGOs define their own indicators based on a logical framework. To date, the EC monitoring systems require the submission of annual narrative progress reports. The Ministry of Public Health has been involved in a review of tender documents and evaluation of proposals, although to a more limited extent than with other models. However, it is envisaged that all procurement responsibilities will be handed over to the Ministry of Public Health in future rounds of funding.

Table 8-3 illustrates the forms that contracting has taken in Afghanistan and details some of the main differences among them. It also highlights some of the changes that donors have made to upcoming rounds of funding in response to greater familiarity with the Afghan context and developments in the health sector. In general, the models have become more similar over time, and newly adopted features have streamlined donor approaches. The World Bank, however, is the only donor with plans to continue incorporating financial bonuses.

Monitoring and Evaluating Systems

For pay for performance to work, performance has to be measured and validated. The value of monitoring and evaluating services delivered has received attention in Afghanistan, and support is being provided by several sources. A new national Health Management Information System (HMIS) has been put in place by the Ministry of Public Health together with USAID's REACH project, and training has been conducted on a national scale to establish systems at the provincial level.

The HMIS represents the national monitoring system that all providers are required to report on, but donors have established additional mechanisms to monitor performance. Some of these are specific to donor activities, and some cover all facilities.

Table 8-3. *Reporting, Monitoring, and Evaluation in Afghanistan, by Donor Program*

USAID	World Bank, Ministry of Public Health	European Commission
Submission of detailed quarterly reports	Submission of quarterly technical and HMIS reports	Submission of annual technical and financial reports
Quarterly monitoring visits (one visit per facility per quarter)	Third-party performance assessment conducted annually nationwide	Submission of quarterly technical and HMIS reports to the Ministry of Public Health
Implementation of fully functional service delivery point	and semiannually in performance-based partnership agreements, Ministry of Public	Ad hoc monitoring visits from European Commission head office in Brussels
Household surveys conducted at baseline, midterm, and end of project by NGOs	Health strengthening mechanism, and three European Commission projects	
Semiannual roundtable meetings	Ad hoc monitoring missions conducted by the Ministry of Public Health and the World Bank	
Semiannual face-to-face meetings	Monthly performance-based partnership agreements coordination meetings and some face-to-face meetings	
	Wide circulation of aide-mémoires documenting mission findings to all stakeholders	

Source: Authors.

The World Bank is funding a large external evaluation program conducted by Johns Hopkins University and the Indian Institute of Health Management Research (IIHMR). This includes four annual assessments of the performance of national health facilities in all thirty-four provinces and three semiannual assessments in eleven provinces covered by World Bank contracts (eight provinces with NGO contracts plus the three MoPH-SM provinces) as well as three provinces covered by EC grants.

Based on the annual assessments, scores on a balanced scorecard are calculated at the provincial level. Details of the components are shown in table 8-4. The

Table 8-4. *Components of the Balanced Scorecard*

Domain	Component	Detail
Patients and community	Patient satisfaction	Patients were asked to rank whether they were satisfied with their visit
	Patient perceptions of quality	Patients were asked to score a range of quality-related items such as courtesy of staff, cleanliness, and availability and cost of drugs. This is a composite index of nine items
	Written community health committee activities	Percent of facilities with a written record of activities
Staff	Health worker satisfaction index	Staff were asked to rank fourteen measures of their own satisfaction such as working relationship with other staff, availability of equipment, and salary. This is a composite index of these fourteen items
	Salary payments current	Whether staff have received their salary within the past month
Capacity for service provision	Equipment functionality index	Presence of key equipment, such as weighing scales for children, thermometer, and sterilizer
	Drug availability index	Presence of five key drugs (Paracetemol, Amoxicillin, Tetracycline eye ointment, ORS packets, and iron tablets)
	Family planning availability index	Presence of family planning supplies
	Lab functionality index	Eleven items to measure the functionality of the facility's laboratory
	Staffing index	Whether the facility had the requisite staff as prescribed by the basic package of health services
	Provider knowledge score	Level of knowledge of providers relevant to their cadre
	Staff received training in last year	Percentage of staff who attended post service training in the last year
	HMIS use index	Availability and upkeep of HMIS
	Clinical guidelines index	Availability of various clinical guidelines

(continued)

Table 8-4. *Components of the Balanced Scorecard (continued)*

Domain	Component	Detail
	Infrastructure index	Appropriate number and condition of rooms
	Patient record index	Maintenance of appropriate patient records
	Facilities having tuberculosis register	Availability of tuberculosis registers
Service provision	Patient-provider care index	Time spent to check a patient
	Proper disposal of sharp objects	Checks for proper disposal of sharp objects
	Average new outpatient visits per month	Number of new patients
	Provision of antenatal care services	Availability of antenatal care services
	Delivery of care according to the basic package of health services	Availability of delivery services
Financial systems	Facilities with user fee guidelines	Availability of user fee guidelines
	Facilities with exemptions	Facilities with exemption mechanisms for poor people
Overall vision	Females as a percent of new outpatients	Females as a percent of new outpatients
	Outpatient visit concentration index	Proportion of poor versus rich using health services
	Patient satisfaction concentration index	Satisfaction of poor versus rich with health services

Source: Ministry of Public Health, Johns Hopkins University, and IIHMR (2004).

scorecard is based on a random sample of health facilities in a province and measures the extent to which their activities are aligned with those prescribed by the basic package of health services. This mechanism is the only independent monitoring and evaluation mechanism in place that documents performance in all provinces, making it a valuable investment for the Ministry of Public Health.

Other monitoring mechanisms include the submission of quarterly narrative, financial, and HMIS reports to the Ministry of Public Health and ad hoc monitoring missions to the field (a World Bank midterm review in mid-2005 and quarterly visits under REACH contracts, for example). USAID introduced the fully functional service delivery point (FFSDP) monitoring tool as a way for NGOs to monitor the level of quality in facilities. It consists of internal and external exercises to monitor improvements in a number of indicators related to quality of care. Many of the indicators are similar to those included in the balanced scorecard.

Table 8-5. *Proportion of Facilities to Population in Afghanistan, 2002–05*

Indicator	Number
Number of provinces	34
Number of health facilities	
Baseline	606
Current	1,050
Population	20,569,020
Ratio of health facilities to population	
Baseline	1:33,993
Current	1:19,560

Source: Authors.

The FFSDP tool aims to encourage NGOs to monitor their own performance. To date, the FFSDP tool has been implemented in 65 percent of REACH facilities, and there are plans to pilot it in four provinces with World Bank and EC contracts, with the possibility of expanding it to the entire country.

Under USAID's REACH project, NGOs are responsible for conducting their own baseline, midterm, and end-of-project household surveys using the lot quality assurance sampling methodology. The surveys collect baseline and subsequent information on ten key health indicators focused on maternal health, reproductive health, and child health. Data have been collected by staff employed by NGOs such as community health workers. Questions have been raised over the reliability of the results given that the NGOs are directly responsible for data collection. REACH has provided close supervision and engaged NGOs in joint analysis to reduce the possibility of falsifying results.

CONTRACTING NGOS

Overall, contracting NGOs has helped to expand service delivery rapidly. Between early 2003 and mid-2006, availability of the basic package of health services has expanded to all thirty-four provinces, nominally covering 82 percent of the population, with only sixteen districts and the centers of some major cities still uncovered. In addition, the proportion of facilities to population has increased from one facility for every 34,000 people to one for every 20,000 people (see table 8-5), and inequities among provinces have been reduced. At baseline, the availability of health facilities ranged from one for every 12,027–92,578 people. By 2005, this gap had been reduced to a range of one facility for every 12,027–26,968 people (Ministry of Public Health 2005). Significant progress has also been made in recruiting and placing female staff in facilities, specifically, a

Figure 8-1. *Change in the Number of Female Clinical Health Workers in Afghanistan, by Province*

Number of female health workers

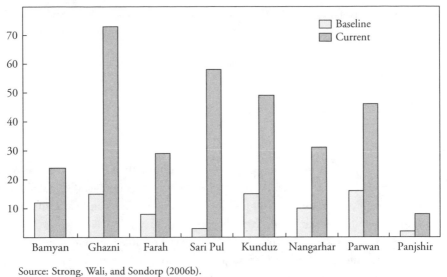

Source: Strong, Wali, and Sondorp (2006b).

300 percent increase within the eight case study locations examined by Strong, Wali, and Sondorp (2005; see figure 8-1).

Promising progress toward reaching health service delivery targets such as immunization coverage (DPT3) and skilled delivery has also been made (see figure 8-2). For example, analysis of HMIS data shows that the number of women delivering in health facilities more than doubled between 2004 and 2005 (see figure 8-3).[1] The proportion of women receiving a first antenatal care visit at least doubled in all approaches (see figure 8-4). Findings from the third-party evaluation show that the number of facilities providing antenatal care in the three MoPH-SM provinces increased from an average of 45 percent to 75 percent between the first annual round of facility-based inspections in 2004 and the first semiannual round in 2005.

1. Because pockets of data in the HMIS database were missing, all data were corrected for under-reporting. Data were analyzed by quarter. If data for one month of the quarter were missing, then the mean of the remaining months in the quarter was calculated. The HMIS database was more incomplete for some donor areas than for others, which necessitated these corrections to allow for valid comparisons of performance across approaches.

Figure 8-2. *DPT3 Coverage in Afghanistan, 2004 and 2005*

Percent

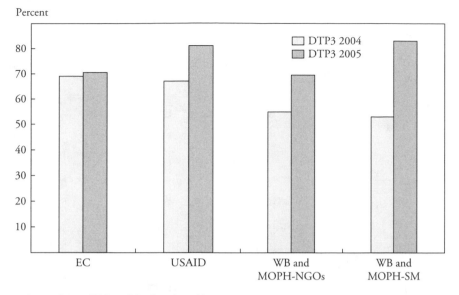

Source: Strong, Wali, and Sondorp (2006a).

Figure 8-3. *Proportion of Deliveries Attended by Skilled Birth Attendants in Afghanistan, Corrected for Underreporting, 2004 and 2005*

Percent

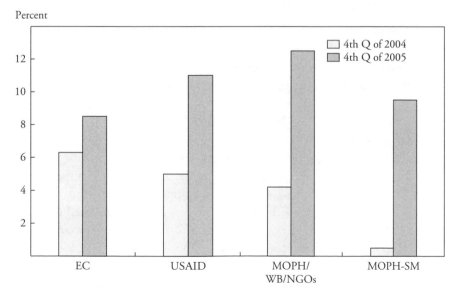

Source: Strong, Wali, and Sondorp (2006a).

Figure 8-4. *Proportion of Pregnant Women Receiving First Antenatal Care Visit in Afghanistan, 2004 and 2005*

Percent

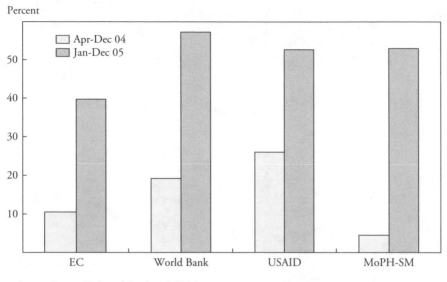

Source: Strong, Wali, and Sondorp (2006a).

PERFORMANCE-BASED PAYMENT

Contracting NGOs has clearly increased the availability and use of the basic package of health services by the Afghan population. It is less clear whether the different donor approaches, and in particular performance-based payment by the World Bank, have influenced the effectiveness of NGOs.

Data

HMIS data show that the number of consultations per person per year has increased steadily over time (see figure 8-5). All donor approaches show the same general trend over 2005, but the MoPH-SM model appears to have outperformed the others. There has been wide interest in the potential for comparing the effectiveness of the different approaches taken by donors using the balanced scorecard data. Figure 8-6 illustrates the mean performance by contracting group according to the balanced scorecard in 2004 and 2005. The net gain in each group was 3.5 (European Commission), 12.2 (World Bank), 10.1 (REACH), and 8.1 (MoPH-SM). World Bank–NGO provinces score the highest, followed by those of USAID, the MoPH-SM, and the European Commission. Bonuses are paid in

Figure 8-5. *Number of Consultations per Person per Year in Afghanistan,*
Corrected for Underreporting

Number of consultations

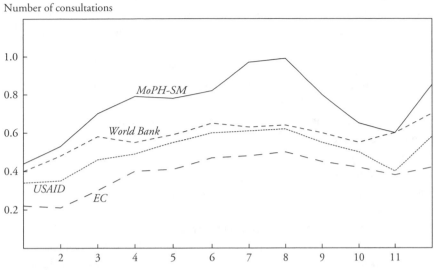

Source: Strong, Wali, and Sondorp (2006a).

Figure 8-6. *Comparative Performance in Afghanistan, by Contracting Group,*
2004 and 2005

Mean score in all domains

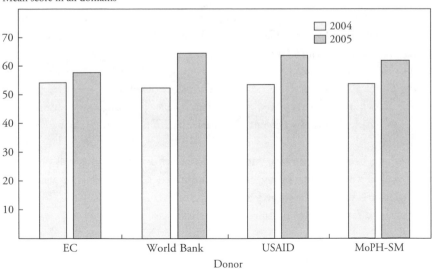

Source: Strong, Wali, and Sondorp (2006a).

the World Bank scheme according to percentage change over time rather than absolute score. The pay-for-performance mechanism appears to be outperforming the other models, but the differences are relatively small.

Results

The balanced scorecard and the HMIS suggest different patterns of achievement for different groups of NGOs. Both sources of information should be interpreted with care. Various factors may influence performance as reflected in the balanced scorecard, and concluding that variations are attributable to pay for performance alone is not possible. Equally, data from the HMIS may not be accurate enough to reflect differences among providers. There are several drawbacks to comparing performance on the basis of an assessment such as the balanced scorecard.

First, the data exclusively reflect services provided at functional facilities. This introduces a bias for provinces that have only a handful of functional facilities in more accessible areas. A province with extremely low and unequal coverage may receive a good score if the few facilities that exist are doing well. For instance, in Zabul and Uruzgan, only four facilities were included in the initial 2004 assessment, yet the provinces were ranked first and fourth of thirty-four (Ministry of Public Health, Johns Hopkins University, and IIHMR 2006), despite the fact that many residents of these provinces had limited, if any, access.

Second, the balanced scorecard was designed primarily to measure performance in province-wide projects funded by the World Bank. As such, interpretation in USAID and some EC provinces is more difficult because one NGO does not necessarily cover an entire province.

Third, balanced scorecard results were not meant to be compared directly across donor approaches. Given that the data do not report the relative starting points in each of the areas or provinces and are not weighted for security and geographic considerations, a 5 percent increase in a difficult setting may be a greater achievement than a 15 percent increase in an easier setting.

Last, the balanced scorecard cannot reflect improvements in access or health outcomes for the broader community.[2] Although these assessments provide some information on access, the information is limited to populations living within the immediate catchment area of functional facilities sampled.

---

2. To address this problem, the Ministry of Public Health, with World Bank funding, is commissioning the same third party to conduct a small national sample household survey to measure a collection of health coverage indicators. Data from this are not yet available.

Similarly, the apparently good performance of the MoPH-SM must be reviewed critically as an example of further contextual confounding factors:

—The three provinces within the MoPH-SM are near Kabul and enjoy good security, creating more favorable circumstances for attracting trained and experienced health staff. For example, several female health providers are transported daily from Kabul to the health facilities in the province where they work (Strong, Wali, and Sondorp 2006a).

—Most facilities were already well established and being run by reputable NGOs when the MoPH-SM took over the provinces.

—The MoPH-SM team has the authority to hire and fire provincial health staff, including the provincial health director, which allows them to create the best circumstances possible for successful implementation.

—The MoPH-SM subcontracts a range of services. In one province, for example, the provincial hospital and several clinics are managed by an NGO. Several components of the basic package of health services, such as community health worker and midwifery training, have also been contracted to NGOs.

Finally, it is clear that the monitoring and evaluation tools being used by different stakeholders produce different results. For example, data on skilled attendance at deliveries for USAID areas vary depending on the source used. HMIS data show that skilled deliveries at the end of 2005 were 11.18 percent of all deliveries, on average (Ministry of Public Health 2005 in Strong, Wali, and Sondorp 2005). USAID's end-of-project household survey shows 22.9 percent for the first two rounds of grants (Ministry of Public Health, Management Sciences for Health 2006). Finally, the balanced scorecard data show that delivery care according to the basic package of health services was 32.5 percent in 2005 (Ministry of Public Health, Johns Hopkins University, and IIHMR 2006). Clearly all these data have confidence intervals that are wider than many of the differences reported for the performance of different models.

The health module of the National Resource Vulnerability Assessment, scheduled to begin in 2007 and designed to produce information on coverage indicators such as immunization at the district level, should prove useful. In addition, the Afghan household survey to be conducted by the Johns Hopkins University and IIHMR may provide complementary information. Accurately measuring performance under different contractual approaches will be a long-term process. Currently, using balanced scorecard data to compare performance between providers and donor models to draw conclusions on their effectiveness may not be appropriate.

However, based on the limited information available at the time of writing, NGOs paid through contracts that incorporate performance-based payments appear to do relatively well. Factors other than the opportunity to earn performance bonuses may be driving this apparent better performance. Another possible contributor to performance is the autonomy and flexibility to use funds in ways that NGO management deems most effective. Input-based reimbursement approaches, by contrast, require accounting for spending on inputs according to a predetermined budget and may limit flexibility to change the mix of inputs. The emphasis by the Ministry of Public Health and donors on monitoring results may also be driving better performance. The perceptions of the different stakeholders shed some light on the various factors that play a role.

Stakeholder Perceptions

Qualitative interviews in the study by Strong, Wali, and Sondorp (2005) explored the perceptions, experiences, and attitudes of donors, the Ministry of Public Health, and NGOs to the idea of using performance bonuses. NGOs were asked about their perceptions regarding performance-based approaches and whether they had spurred changes in the way they operated.

Although some providers felt that pay for performance was too early to introduce in the Afghan context, others felt that a more explicit focus on results was having a good impact on their performance by encouraging NGOs to work harder. A number of NGOs, for example, cited that difficulties related to obtaining needed inputs—such as drugs and supplies, health professionals, training, and equipment—limited their ability to achieve the desired outcomes. Additionally, it was thought that although the overall idea of pay for performance was good, the timing was not right.

The focus on performance has encouraged NGOs to become more decentralized and to improve their monitoring capacity. Some felt that the new emphasis on performance motivated useful management and organizational changes that strengthened their capacity. Changes in structure included the addition of HMIS officers and provincial monitors to allow for closer tracking of progress toward targets. In general, NGOs felt that their organizations had become more decentralized and that this had had a positive impact on performance.

Many interviewees operating under the World Bank model commented that mission findings were extremely useful and that feedback had had a positive influence on their performance. According to one NGO manager, the number of patient consultations increased four times after receiving guidance from a World Bank mission.

USAID-funded NGOs implementing the FFSDP tool also described significant improvements in performance. Interviews with REACH NGOs revealed that the FFSDP tool allowed them to improve the quality of services. It was also suggested that unannounced quarterly monitoring visits to facilities put greater emphasis on performance.

Interviews showed that the most favored aspect of the World Bank approach was the lump-sum contract. The financial flexibility this permitted created more freedom for implementation and responding to changes at the field level. The prospect of obtaining a financial bonus seemed secondary to the lump-sum contract, which represented a new way of doing business for most NGOs involved. Some of the larger NGOs remarked that easy access to funding from other external sources meant that there was no pressure to obtain the 10 percent bonus provided through the scheme.

Another NGO commented that any decisions on how the bonus funds would be used would be determined by their main office and that they were sure that field staff would receive no direct benefit, meaning that the bonus was not really a source of motivation. They felt that if they knew they would receive some personal benefit, then it might serve as an incentive. These views, however, were obtained before bonuses were awarded. Anecdotal evidence collected after the study showed that field staff benefited from performance bonuses, which may help to change the perceptions of this approach.

NGOs that received bonuses showed considerable pride in the outcome. Funds usually were spent on small luxuries for clinics, such as heaters for the staff, and for staff bonuses. It is unclear, however, whether it was the money, the sense of being rewarded for good performance, or both that pleased staff.

Some NGOs cited fear of failure as a more prominent motivator than the performance bonus. Interviews with NGOs operating under the World Bank and REACH schemes revealed that they also felt under pressure to perform. When asked about penalties for poor performance, most World Bank and USAID NGOs said that their contracts would be terminated and their reputations tarnished. By the later stages of fieldwork, all NGOs were aware that national monitoring mechanisms were in place and understood that their performance would be compared with that of other NGOs across the country.

REACH representatives felt that the design and specifications of the grant could improve performance without financial bonuses and have a sustained impact on the organizations and their employees as well. For example, REACH grant requirements include submission of HMIS reports and recruitment of female community health workers. As a result, 98 percent of REACH-supported facilities are submitting HMIS reports and 53 percent of community health workers are female. Workshops on a number of different topics, such as training for illiterate women, have helped REACH grantees to satisfy grant requirements. Another also saw monitoring as a key part of the process of improving performance, without the need for financial incentives. It was claimed that the REACH approach has helped to increase transparency and reduce fraud in the NGOs.

A potential drawback of the pay-for-performance approach has been identified as the tendency to become overly focused on targets. Some stakeholders expressed concern that strong incentives to improve in certain areas of service delivery would weaken the focus on overall quality of care. This was raised by one NGO where the overarching concern was that the new payment arrangements were pushed through very quickly and that this might have an impact on how lasting some of these positive changes would be.

Financial freedom opens the door for NGOs to accumulate funds not spent on project activities. This was of some concern in various parts of the Ministry of Public Health. Under a lump-sum contract, budgets of the winning bid cannot be negotiated, and if organizations spend less than what was budgeted to reach performance targets, they can, in theory, keep the surplus. Although the World Bank has made a few exceptions for budget negotiations, the ministry is still concerned about how the NGO can accrue profit but not allocate any financial benefit for the purchaser. These fears have been quelled to some extent by clauses in World Bank contracts to the effect that any surplus funds must be used for continuing project activities.

Conclusions

We have briefly described the various contractual approaches being used in Afghanistan and considered whether there is evidence on the effects of performance-based payment. What evidence does exist supports the idea that payment for performance has encouraged stronger performance among NGO service providers. It would appear that both World Bank and Ministry of Health provinces are performing very well and better than those providers not receiving a pay-for-performance incentive. However, we have also identified a number of alternative explanations for why this may be the case. These reasons are related both to the way in which performance has been measured (measurement bias) and underlying differences in the provinces in each group (selection bias).

Additional issues related to the implementation of pay for performance in a fragile, postconflict setting should be raised. The first is a question of the degree to which some NGOs are able to respond to the types of incentives presented by a pay-for-performance approach. The pay-for-performance approach is predicated on an idea that, given proper incentives, providers can improve their performance. For some NGOs in Afghanistan, the external constraints in which they operate may mean that this is not the case. It may lead NGOs to fail to bid for the most difficult areas for service delivery.

To better understand the potential impact of pay for performance in Afghanistan, it is also necessary to understand the extent to which field-level workers and managers are aware of the targets that have been set. Several factors are of interest here. First, one donor noted that NGOs were taking time to understand the concept of a fixed budget and the measurement of results. Second, in the REACH project, NGOs spoke of the beneficial effects of both setting and monitoring targets, without the need for a financial bonus. Third, some NGOs appeared to be uncomfortable with the idea of being rewarded financially because it did not fit with their humanitarian mandate. Last, the World Bank contract design—lump-sum contracts with flexibility—received very favorable feedback overall. For example, one NGO that was initially strongly opposed to the concept of performance-based partnership agreements converted completely to the new way of doing business. Indeed, several of the NGO representatives interviewed who have experience with all three donor approaches are ardent supporters of pay for performance and suggest that it has stimulated positive changes in how they work.

Afghanistan's experiment with pay for performance is still in its very earliest days. It is important to watch the results over the next few years with care, but also to be aware of the difficulty of isolating the effect of pay for performance without a randomized study design. It is important to note both the similarities and differences in using pay for performance in a postconflict setting compared to a more stable health system. Some issues appear to be the same, such as the strong incentives pay for performance gives to achieve certain target indicators, but in a postconflict setting, external constraints may hinder providers from responding to pay-for-performance incentives appropriately. Similarly, the motives of NGOs that work in a humanitarian setting may be less influenced by the promise of financial gain.

References

Bartlett, L. A., S. Mawji, S. Whitehead, C. Crouse, S. Dalil, D. Ionete, and P. Salama. 2005. "Where Giving Birth Is a Forecast of Death: Maternal Mortality in Four Districts in Afghanistan, 1999–2002." *Lancet* 365 (9462): 864–70.

Fleck, Fiona. 2004. "Pre-Election Insecurity in Afghanistan Hampers Health Service Delivery." *British Medical Journal* 329 (7463): 420.

Ministry of Public Health. 2005. HMIS Health Management Information System. Kabul.

Ministry of Public Health, Johns Hopkins University, and IIHMR (Indian Institute of Health Management Research). 2004. "Afghanistan Health Sector Balanced Scorecard: National and Provincial Results." Kabul.

———. 2006. "Afghanistan Health Sector Balanced Scorecard, 2004 and 2005." Kabul.

Ministry of Public Health, Management Sciences for Health. 2002. "Afghanistan National Health Resources Assessment." Kabul.

———. 2006. "REACH Baseline and End-of-Project Household Surveys: Comparative Results." Kabul.

Strong, Lesley, Abdul Wali, and Egbert Sondorp. 2005. "Health Policy in Afghanistan: Two Years of Rapid Change." London: London School of Hygiene and Tropical Medicine. (www.lshtm.ac.uk/hpu/conflict/files/publications/file_33.pdf [October 2008].)

———. 2006a. *Contracting Health Services in Afghanistan: A Comparison of Donor Models and Perceptions.* Draft report. London: London School of Hygiene and Tropical Medicine (September).

———. 2006b. *Contracting Health Services in Afghanistan: A Summary of the Research and Case Profiles.* Draft report. London: London School of Hygiene and Tropical Medicine (September).

9

Haiti:
Going to Scale with a Performance
Incentive Model

Rena Eichler, Paul Auxila, Uder Antoine,
and Bernateau Desmangles

Highlights

Rewarding NGOs for increasing access to a package of basic services and paying them
for achieving population-based performance targets can result in significant increases in
essential services such as immunizations and assisted deliveries.

Paying NGOs for results strengthens institutional capacity to deliver services from the
bottom up.

Changes in the design throughout the six years offer lessons for other contexts.

Paying for performance in Haiti is part of a package of interventions in a bilateral health project funded by the U.S. Agency for International Development (USAID) and implemented by Management Sciences for Health that aims to increase coverage and quality of health services. Starting in 1999, payment to contracted nongovernmental organizations (NGOs) changed from simple reimbursement for documented expenditures to payment partly conditional on targets being reached. Remarkable improvements in key health indicators have been achieved over the six years that performance-based payment has been phased in. Now reaching 2.7 million people, NGOs in the project network provide essential services to the Haitian population in the complicated context of violence, poverty, and limited government leadership. The experience in Haiti contributes to understanding whether paying for results works and provides important lessons for the design and implementation of other efforts.

Haiti is one of the poorest and most vulnerable countries in the world: 80 percent of its rural population survives on less than $1 per day (Collymore 2004). Life expectancy at birth is estimated at fifty-three years, infant mortality is 80 per 1,000 live births, and the maternal mortality ratio is 523 per 100,000 live births, seven times higher than in the Dominican Republic (PAHO 2007). According to the Pan American Health Organization, approximately 40 percent of the population has no access to basic health care services. Chronic malnutrition is estimated to affect 25 percent of children under five, and acute respiratory infections and diarrhea cause half of the deaths of young children. Compounding poor child and maternal health is the reality that Haiti has the largest number of people living with HIV/AIDS in the Caribbean, with estimated prevalence between 2.5 and 11.9 percent of the population between fifteen and forty-nine years of age.

In 1995 concern about these indicators and the inability of the Haitian government to ensure access to basic health services motivated USAID to fund a project to contract NGOs to deliver essential services, enhance the capacity of the government to oversee the health sector, and strengthen health service organizations. Immediate needs at the time were critical health services, including maternal and child health, reproductive health, and family planning services. Support was provided to develop public sector–led local health organizing committees, which had the mandate to develop district plans to ensure access to an essential package of services by coordinating public and NGO providers.

Following competitive tenders, USAID awarded management of this three-phase (1995–99, 2000–04, 2005–07) project to Management Sciences for Health, a U.S.-based NGO that strengthens health services in developing countries. USAID included a contractual requirement in the initial phase that specified a shift in payment terms to NGOs from expenditure-based reimbursement to output-based payment. Initially, NGOs were reimbursed for documented expenditures up to a ceiling that was essentially a negotiated budget. The vision of the project was eventually to pay NGOs based on services provided (outputs). This shift was envisioned to occur when NGO capacity could ensure both accountability for results and responsible management of U.S. government funds.

Management Sciences for Health piloted a change in payment based partly on performance, with three NGOs responsible for providing services to roughly half a million people in the final year of the first phase. Promising results led USAID and Management Sciences for Health to integrate payment for results into future phases. Subsequent phases progressively added additional NGOs and experimented with changes in design and implementation. By 2006, all NGOs supported by the program were involved in the strategy, which is now being adapted to fund the public sector. Presented here are six years of experience implementing payment for performance in the challenging Haitian context with lessons learned throughout the process of refining and experimenting with the approach.

Why was improved performance thought to be possible? A 1997 population-based survey found that performance of the NGOs financed by the project was extremely uneven. Some, for example, achieved vaccination coverage of only 7 percent of the target population, but others reached 70 percent; one NGO taught only 44 percent of mothers about oral rehydration therapy (ORT), while another taught 80 percent (Eichler, Auxila, and Pollock 2001).

That some NGOs were performing adequately indicated that improvements were possible for others too. Project staff hypothesized that part of the reason for poor performance was a payment system that placed too much emphasis on transparent documentation and not enough on results. To change this, a new approach was piloted that switched from reimbursing expenditures to payment based partially on the attainment of targets, complemented by technical assistance and data validation.

The Pilot (1999)

The three NGOs chosen to pilot performance-based payment—Centres pour le Développement et la Santé, Comité Bienfaisance de Pignon, and Save the Children—were perceived to have demonstrated the leadership and institutional capacity needed to respond to the new system and were committed to participating in a pilot that linked payment to what they also valued: health results. Believing that it would be important for the NGOs to view the change in payment as advantageous, the project adopted a collaborative approach to design, negotiations, and implementation. The NGOs were invited to participate in meetings and asked their views about participating in the pilot. Because the meetings were held after contracts for the 1999 funding cycle were signed, the NGOs were willing to renegotiate only if the proposed contract had the potential for more funding. Agreement was therefore reached on a model that imposed some financial risk but also offered the potential for more funding (Eichler 2002).[1]

---

1. This is an example of the type of compromise that was needed to be able to move forward.

Table 9-1. *Performance Indicators and Relative Weights in Haiti*

Indicator	Target	Relative weight
Percentage of mothers using oral rehydration solution to treat cases of children with diarrhea	15 percent increase	10 percent of bonus
Full vaccination coverage for children ages birth to eleven months	10 percent increase	20 percent of bonus
At least three prenatal visits	20 percent increase	10 percent of bonus
Reduction in the level of discontinuation rate for injectable and oral contraceptives	25 percent reduction	20 percent of bonus
Number of institutional service delivery points with at least four modern methods of family planning and number of outreach points with at least three or more modern methods	All institutional service delivery points with four or more; 50 percent of outreach points with three or more	20 percent of bonus
Reduction in average waiting time before providing attention to a child (in hours and minutes from arrival to beginning of attention)	50 percent reduction	10 percent of bonus
Participation in establishment of local community health units and coordination with the Ministry of Health	Defined by each local health organizing committee	10 percent of bonus

Source: Authors.

The NGOs agreed on a new contract that would pay 95 percent of the budget established under the existing expenditure-based reimbursement contract and including the possibility of a bonus of as much as 10 percent of the budget. NGOs were thus assuming the risk of losing 5 percent of the agreed budget if they did not reach targets, but they stood to gain an additional 5 percent if they did (Eichler, Auxila, and Pollock 2001).

Seven performance indicators and targets were defined, and NGOs could receive a predefined percentage of the potential bonus for achieving the target increase in each indicator (see table 9-1). Five indicators related to improving health impact, one related to increasing consumer satisfaction by reducing waiting time, and one related to improving coordination with the Ministry of Health. Two of the indicators of health impact were related to family planning: availability of modern methods and reduction in the rate of discontinuation. The latter was chosen to address findings from a series of focus groups suggesting that new family planning acceptors frequently discontinued use because of side effects and poor counseling. The goal was to improve the quality of care. Each NGO separately negotiated performance targets for each indicator, and payment for reaching each target was all or nothing.[2]

Measurement

To ensure that indicators accurately represented performance and to ensure credibility of the pilot, the project contracted an independent survey research firm—Institut Haitien de l'Enfance (IHE)—to measure baseline and end-of-pilot performance. IHE followed the standard World Health Organization cluster sampling methodology to sample households to establish baseline measures and results and used immunization cards and reports from caretakers. The percentage of women using ORT for diarrhea was determined by exit interviews in service delivery institutions. Coverage of pregnant women with three or more prenatal visits was determined through household interviews and sample records. Discontinuation rates for oral contraceptives and injectables were determined by reviewing family planning registers. Average waiting time was determined by measuring waiting times in a sample of institutions at different intervals.

The project had to rely on official government projections about population figures in service areas, however imperfect, in the absence of a recent census. These rough figures for the number of each target population group, such as children younger than one and pregnant women, are the denominator of the performance measures, which are expressed as a percentage of a priority population group that receives the intended services.

Results

Table 9-2 presents baseline measures, targets, and results for each participating NGO. Most striking were the increases in immunization coverage beyond performance targets for all three NGOs. In two of the three service areas, the proportion of mothers who reported using ORT and using it correctly increased. Performance in the number of prenatal visits and reduction in the discontinuation rates for oral contraceptives and injectables was relatively weak, although the availability of modern contraceptive methods increased substantially.

---

2. Lack of consensus among the USAID community about whether this indicator complied with the Tiahrt Amendment (see chapter 3) caused the project to eliminate this indicator in subsequent periods.

Table 9-2. *Results from Performance-Based Payment Pilot in Haiti*[a]

Indicator	NGO 1			NGO 2			NGO 3		
	Baseline	*Target*	*Results*	*Baseline*	*Target*	*Results*	*Baseline*	*Target*	*Results*
Immunization coverage	40	44	79	49	54	69	35	38	73
Three or more prenatal care services	32	38	36	49	59	44	18	21	16
Family planning discontinuation	32	24	43	43	32	30	26	20	12
Use of ORT	43	50	47	56	64	50	56	64	86
Correct use of ORT	71	80	81	53	59	26	61	67	74
Institutions with four or more modern family planning services	6	9	9	2	5	5	0	5	5

Source: Eichler, Auxila, and Pollock (2001).

a. Baseline is as of September 1999; results are as of April 2000.

This pilot demonstrates that it is not necessary to get all the details right from the outset to be effective. One of many examples of learning and change to the performance-based payment approach in Haiti is that two indicators were found to be invalid and thus eliminated. The indicator of waiting time was dropped from the scheme because people often chose to wait rather than return from long distances for laboratory test results; patients saw long waiting times at one NGO as an indicator of quality rather than poor service. The bonus associated with the indicator that measured community participation and collaboration with the Ministry of Health was given to each NGO. Although all agreed that participation and collaboration were important, a measurable and verifiable indicator was difficult to determine.

All three NGOs received more revenue than they would have under the previous expenditure-based scheme, although none received the bonus for all indicators. Because performance was measured by examining a sample of the population, confidence intervals made it difficult to determine whether results were statistically significant. When the results attained fell below the target but were within one confidence interval, the NGO was given the bonus. This challenge was one of the reasons the method of measuring performance was refined in subsequent phases.

Reactions

NGOs supported continuing performance-based payment, believing that focusing on results inspired them to question and experiment with their models of service delivery. They strongly endorsed the expanded managerial and budgetary flexibility and the increased motivation of staff, who became more attentive to their organization's objectives and more innovative about achieving them, for example, by increasing community participation. Everyone emphasized the need for good data and information for decisionmaking. Over the course of the pilot, modifications were made, and the three NGOs shared what they learned.

To achieve performance targets, two of the three created bonus schemes for staff. One implemented a bonus scheme for local organizations with whom they collaborated. Another did the same for community health agents, cutting their salary in half and reserving the rest for bonuses tied to performance. But the poor results from transferring this degree of risk to relatively low-paid staff led the NGOs to increase the fixed proportion of payment and reduce the proportion of bonuses. One reported that imposing excessive financial risk was demotivating. All wished to allocate a proportion of any earned bonus to improving clinic infrastructure.

Performance-based payment did motivate NGOs to request technical assistance. Being demand driven, such assistance proved particularly effective at strengthening NGO institutional capacity. It also helped the project to be more strategic and cost-effective in providing support aligned more directly with the results to be achieved.

An Evolving Approach (2000–06)

Encouraged by pilot results and NGO endorsement, performance-based payment was adopted as a core strategy in 2000. Figure 9-1 presents the gradual addition of NGOs into performance-based payment during the eight contract periods of the project, beginning with the 1999 pilot year. The 2005 period shows a radical shift from twelve to twenty-five NGOs being paid based on performance and a concurrent reduction in the number of expenditure-based NGOs from fifteen to two. Through the period, changes were made to how performance-based payments were designed and implemented to increase effectiveness and adapt to changing realities, such as the interpretation of donor regulations and recalculation of NGO target populations. By the end of 2005, this project supported delivery of basic

Figure 9-1. *Scaling Up Payment for Performance*

Number of NGOs

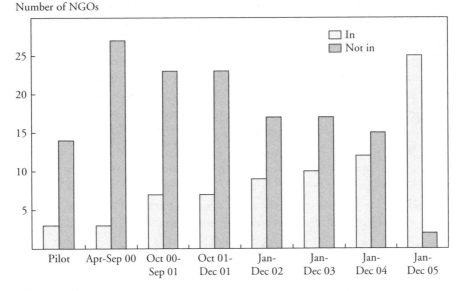

Source: Authors.

health services to 2.7 million people by contracted NGOs, with results reaching twice the national average for some indicators.

What Changed and Why?

The seven contract periods that followed the initial pilot cover four distinct phases, each of which introduced changes in design and implementation.

—In phase one (April 2000 to December 2001), expensive community-based surveys gave way to self-reporting by NGOs, complemented by audits from an independent firm.

—In phase two (January 2002 to December 2003), the number of NGOs under performance-based payment increased to nine, and changes were made in performance indicators. Payment was linked to performance on a randomly selected group of technical output and management indicators.

—In phase three (2004), two packages of indicators were defined to serve each priority population group, with either one being randomly chosen for evaluation.

—In phase four (2005), the number of NGOs paid based on results jumped from twelve to twenty-five as a consequence of project efforts to make all NGO partners ready to be paid partially on results. Uniform performance targets were set for all NGOs, regardless of their baselines, and the amount of payment at risk increased.

What follows is a more detailed discussion of how NGOs were selected to be included in performance-based payment, the performance indicators used, how performance was evaluated, the payment terms used, and the reasons for the changes in design introduced in each phase.

SELECTION

Standardized tools were developed and refined to assess readiness and, throughout 2004, NGOs were selected based on this assessment process. In phase one, the project developed an institutional assessment guideline with technical assistance from a local subcontractor, Group Croissance. Under it, NGOs needed to provide a minimum package of services and have a defined target population, sound technical performance, a record of good audit reports and financial review results, adequate monitoring, data, and management information systems and capabilities, as well as the expressed commitment of senior management to participate under changed terms. (There was no predetermined number of NGOs that would be eligible to be paid based on performance.) In phases two and three, the assessment tool was further refined. In phase four, all NGOs in the project network were paid based on performance, eliminating the need for assessments of institutional readiness.

INDICATORS

In addition to technical output indicators, management indicators were added and refined over the phases. In all cases, the previous period's result was the next period's baseline. Targets for the coming year, however, were sometimes set at lower than baseline because of factors such as migration, unreliable population figures, and political instability.

In phase one, the availability of modern methods of family planning was eliminated because the goal was so easily achieved, making it a weak indicator of improved service. The other indicators of technical service output were the same as those used during the pilot. The indicator of reduced waiting time for child visits was dropped because of its poor indication of quality, and the indicator specifying collaboration with the local public sector was dropped because of difficulty in measurement. Six performance indicators were included:

—Full immunization coverage for children under one,
—Three or more prenatal care visits,
—Reduced discontinuation of modern family planning methods,
—Postnatal care visits,
—Assisted deliveries by trained birth attendant, and
—Percentage of children weighed and enrolled in nutritional recuperation programs.

In phase two, management indicators were added to ensure that paying more attention to short-term improvements was not resulting in the neglect of key management functions and investments in needed capacity. Special efforts were directed at promoting the long-term sustainability of NGOs:

—Strengthening drug and commodities management,
—Ensuring timely and correct submission of technical and financial reports,
—Encouraging application or adaptation of guidelines developed by the project in financial management, human resources management, and essential drugs logistics,
—Ensuring that management audit recommendations were addressed,
—Strengthening organizational structure, and
—Promoting the use of the cost and revenue analysis tool.

In addition, the family planning target of reducing discontinuation was eliminated because of lack of clarity about whether this complied with U.S. government regulations.

In phase three, the list of technical indicators was expanded and organized into two "packages" covering different target population groups. In phase four, the same performance benchmarks were applied to all NGOs to streamline monitoring and payment, and the financial risk and possible awards in payment were increased. Targets were the same for NGOs starting with a low as well as a high baseline because considerable technical assistance had been provided to all. It was found, however, that uniform targets placed significant stress on low-performing NGOs. In 2006 the project began to reassess and revise its use of customized performance targets. The overall results have been outstanding.

MEASUREMENT

NGOs report results that are verified by random audits, thus reducing the costs of verification. In phase one, technical output indicators were no longer measured by an independent firm. Performance was instead self-reported by NGOs and confirmed through random audits. Any concerns about inflated results proved unfounded. In phase two, the project randomly chose indicators from an expanded list to ensure that NGOs did not neglect any essential services. Performance on management indicators was assessed by both an independent local firm and the project team. In phase three, one of two packages of indicators was randomly chosen for evaluation. In phase four, an independent firm verified the accuracy of NGO-reported technical indicators through random audits, and the project team assessed management indicators.

PAYMENT

The payment instrument is a fixed-price contract plus an award fee. Types of indicators, the approach to choosing the indicators, and the amount of financial risk imposed on NGOs changed throughout the phases. In phase one, the payment instrument was a fixed-price contract plus award fee, with roughly 10 percent of payment "at risk," conditional on performance targets. In phase two, a new feature was incorporated: 5 percent of the award fee (the withhold) was tied to achieving performance on management indicators, and the other 5 percent (the bonus) was tied to health results. In phase three, these contract terms were maintained. Although the potential reward for health results was reduced in comparison with phase one, uncertainty about which indicators would be chosen was introduced,

Table 9-3. *Performance Benchmarks, Targets, and Payment Links in Haiti, 2005*

Benchmark	Proportion of annual negotiated budget
Sign contract	10 percent
Submit annual action plan	15 percent
Submit monthly reports	1/12 of 10 percent of approved budget each month
Recommendations on financial system strengthening applied	No money
Quarterly requests for payment submitted	March 1, 2005: 20 percent; July 1, 2005: 20 percent; October 1, 2005: 13 percent; November 30: 6 percent
80 percent of children under one completely vaccinated (same target for all NGOs)	1.5 percent
50 percent of pregnant women receiving three prenatal care visits (same target for all NGOs)	1.5 percent

Random choice of one indicator from the following list:
   50 percent of children under five weighed according to guidelines
   63 percent of deliveries are assisted by a trained attendant
   44 percent of women with new births receive a home postnatal care visit
   50 percent of pregnant women are tested for HIV during a prenatal care visit
   75 percent of new positive TB patients are also tested for HIV
	3 percent

Timely submission of quarterly reports to the project	No money
Supervision system with specified criteria in place	No money
Additional bonus if *all* previous targets are met	6 percent
Maximum possible	106 percent of negotiated budget

Source: Authors.

weakening the incentive associated with the payment approach. In phase four, NGO payments were linked to a specific milestone in program implementation, a contract management function, or a service delivery result. Table 9-3 lists the 2005 performance targets and the portion of the budget associated with each indicator.

MANAGEMENT

The project has nine staff members who are part of one of three administrative units responsible for finance, contracting, and information monitoring.

Table 9-4. *Finance, Contract Administration, and Monitoring in Haiti: Staffing, Functions, and Interactions*

Issue	Finance	Contract administration	Monitoring
Staffing	Accounts payable, financial analyst, chief accountant, and chief of finance	Contract administrator, program assistant	Monitoring unit chief, data operator, data analyst
Functions	Process payments, monitor implementation of audit recommendations, part of the team to negotiate contract terms	Prepare contract, request USAID approvals, authorize payments in accordance with contractual clauses (based on the predefined deliverables), part of the team to negotiate contract terms	Depending on the weaknesses identified, provide field-based technical assistance for data collecting and reporting, review and validate the data reporting, process and analyze data, produce information for monitoring and measuring the accomplishment of objectives
Interaction	Ensure constant availability of funds to process payment requests received, ensure that payment is authorized by contract administration	Ensure that technical reports are acceptable to the monitoring unit, ensure that payment requests are transferred to the finance team	After review and acceptance, send a copy of the technical reports to contract administration to process payment
Technical assistance	Technical assistance cuts across the three functions. It is provided on request and based on field visits and assessments made by the project technical team. Based on the information generated by monitoring and evaluation unit on a quarterly basis, meetings are organized with the technical team to discuss results, provide formal feedback to NGOs, and assist NGOs to make programmatic decisions to improve performance of the institutions.		

Source: Authors.

Table 9-4 describes the staffing and functions of these units and shows how they interact with other units in the project, integrating these administrative functions into the technical strategies of the project. This point is extremely important, as clear links with the team that provides technical assistance facilitates strategic planning of technical assistance interventions and timely support to the NGOs.

Table 9-5. *Demographic and Health Survey and Project Results in Haiti*
Percent

Source of data	Immunization	Prenatal	Deliveries	Postnatal
Demographic and Health Survey, 2000	34	29	58	9
Project				
April–Sept 2000	63	47	56	n.a.
October 2000–September 2001	80	46	65	11
October–December 2001[a]	87	91	99	38
2002	65	50	64	34
2003	91	41	57	37
2004	92	48	63	42
2005	100	60	77	50
Demographic and Health Survey, 2005	41.3	84.5[b]	60	n.a.

Source: Authors.
n.a. Not available.
a. Two-month contract period.
b. The 2005 Demographic and Health Survey measures percentage of pregnant women receiving at least one prenatal care visit.

RESULTS

NGOs in the project network performed considerably better than all of Haiti in a sample of four key indicators: full immunization coverage, prenatal care, assisted deliveries, and postnatal care. A comparison between 2000 and preliminary 2005 Demographic and Health Survey data for Haiti and aggregate performance of the NGOs in the project network during each of the post-pilot contract periods indicates considerably better performance in three indicators and slightly better performance in one indicator, as shown in table 9-5. Overall project performance was best in 2005 when the majority of NGOs were under performance-based payment.

The Evidence

To understand whether performance-based payment arrangements are associated with better results, a series of comparisons and econometric tests were run. A number of confounders that complicate the interpretation of simple comparisons are important to bear in mind:

—First, the two are not necessarily equivalent. NGOs were not selected randomly but, instead, were chosen because they were perceived to be ready to graduate into the new payment regime. One explanation for better performance among those in the program could be that they were already better performers.

—Second, because NGOs want to graduate to performance-based payment arrangements, the incentive effect may improve performance early and color the results of the earlier period.

—Third, recalculating NGO baselines and targets skews year-to-year comparisons. Because population figures forming the denominator of NGO targets and performance results are both imperfect and in flux, changes in performance from year to year may be driven partly by a newly calculated population in an NGO catchment area.

—Fourth, performance-based NGOs aggressively negotiate for feasible baselines and targets because payment is affected by whether targets are reached. Their counterparts, by contrast, tend to accept passively whatever targets are proposed.

—Fifth, performance data are likely to be more reliable for performance-based NGOs because of audits.

—Last, environmental factors may explain the changed performance, as may the circumstances in a given contract period, such as the security situation or whether vaccines are available.

To understand whether being paid based on results is associated with better performance, data for the four indicators—full immunization coverage, prenatal care, assisted deliveries, and postnatal care—were compared for each period. NGOs were separated on the basis of performance-based and expenditure-based reimbursement, and a mean was then calculated to establish the average performance for each group. The number of NGOs changes in each period as some graduate to performance-based payment arrangements. This number also varies depending on the indicator, because not all NGOs provide the full package of services. In 2005 most were paid based on performance, and only two were paid based on cost. Table 9-6 shows the number of NGOs in each group in each contract period, which are the data used for the calculations in figures 9-2 through 9-5.[3]

NGOs in performance-based payment arrangements do better with immunization coverage, on average, than those under expenditure-based reimbursement

3. Not all NGOs are included because either they were not evaluated on the specified indicators or their reported performance when "not in" performance-based payment was more than 20 percentage points higher than the highest performance value recorded for an NGO during a period in performance-based payment. These NGOs were dropped because of concerns about data quality in the absence of an audit.

Table 9-6. *Number of NGOs in Performance-Based Payments Schemes in Haiti*

Time period	Immuni-zation		Prenatal		Deliveries		Postnatal	
	In	Out	In	Out	In	Out	In	Out
April–September 2000	3	9	4	10	n.a.	n.a.	n.a.	n.a.
October 2000–September 2001	7	10	7	11	6	8	5	7
October–December 2001	7	10	7	11	6	8	5	9
January–December 2002	7	9	9	10	8	7	8	12
January–December 2003	8	11	9	12	8	12	8	15
January–December 2004	9	12	10	13	9	14	10	15
January–December 2005	19	2	21	1	22	1	23	1

Source: Authors.
n.a. Not available.

in every period except 2003 (see figure 9-2). In 2002 and 2003 the potential reward was reduced and the uncertainty about which indicators might be chosen for assessment increased, possibly resulting in this deterioration in performance. Overall performance improved substantially over the period, suggesting that the focus on performance and associated award contributed to the results. NGOs

Figure 9-2. *Immunization Comparison*

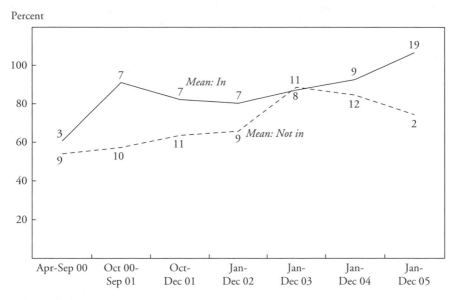

Source: Authors.

Figure 9-3. *Prenatal Comparison*

Percent

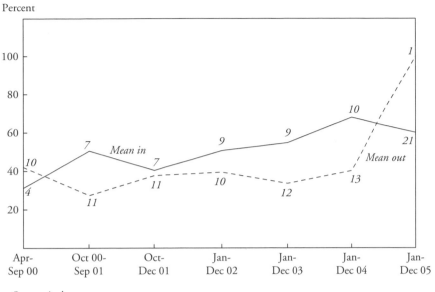

under performance-based payment exhibit consistently better results than their counterparts, except in the initial contract and final period, although the strong performance among those with expenditure-based arrangements was of one NGO, whereas the performance-based mean was of twenty-one NGOs. Results for performance-based NGOs almost doubled between the first contract period and 2005. In deliveries assisted by a trained attendant, performance-based NGOs outperformed expenditure-based NGOs throughout the five years (see figures 9-3 and 9-4). Overall performance for performance-based NGOs improved only slightly, from 78.5 to 80 percent. This change is more striking, however, in light of the fact that only six NGOs were included in the initial period and twenty-two were included in the final period. In postnatal care, performance of both groups improved dramatically, from 21 percent initially to 57 percent in 2005 (see figure 9-5).

As a point of comparison with previous years, 2005 is ideal because almost all NGOs were by then performance based. In previous years, NGOs were selected based on readiness; thus if the results of performance-based NGOs were better than those of expenditure-based NGOs, those results could be attributed to something other than performance incentives. In 2005 this selection problem no longer

Figure 9-4. *Assisted Delivery Comparison*

Percent

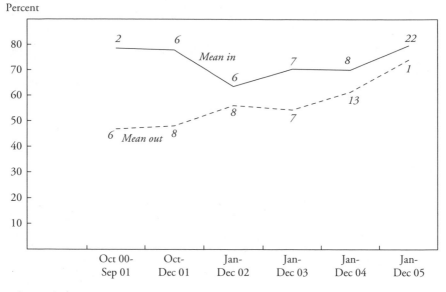

Source: Authors.

Figure 9-5. *Postnatal Comparison*

Percent

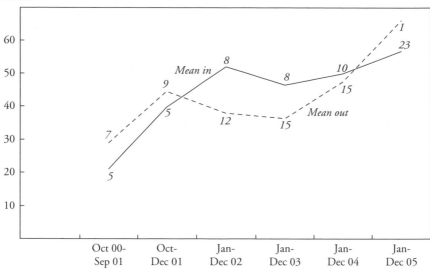

Source: Authors.

Table 9-7. *Average Change in Performance in Haiti*

Indicator	Immunizations	Prenatal	Deliveries	Postnatal
Number up	11	10	10	16
Number down	4	6	5	4
Stayed the same	1	1	1	
Total NGOs that exhibited changes[a]	16	17	16	20
Average percentage change in performance of NGOs in the year prior to, and first year in, performance-based payment[b]	20	15	20	12
Average percentage change in performance for the project over all contract periods[c]	6.2	2.2	3	7.8

Source: Authors.

a. NGOs under performance-based payment for the entire period were not included.

b. For each NGO, changes in performance were calculated from the year prior to entrance into performance-based payment and the first year in performance-based payment. This period differs by NGO and spans all contract periods. For cases when NGOs entered and exited twice, the final contract period was used.

c. Changes in project-level performance between each contract period were calculated, and the overall average change in performance is presented for comparison.

existed, and performance was even better. Although one year of experience is not enough to conclude that tying financial incentives to performance contributes to results, the evidence is supportive.

Another way to explore the question is to compare an NGO's performance on specific indicators in the year before performance-based payment was introduced and in the first year after that. Table 9-7 shows this average change on the four indicators, and the change for performance-based NGOs is considerably larger than that of the project NGOs as a whole. The average jump between the year before and the first year after suggests that at least part of the improvement is driven by the change in payment method.

Regression results that control for NGO-specific characteristics and contract period effects indicate that being paid based on performance is associated with large and significant increases in immunization coverage and assisted deliveries.

To further examine whether payment based on performance is associated with improved results, panel regressions were run covering eight contract periods. Regressions adjust for selection bias arising from characteristics specific to an individual NGO and for contract period effects. The regressions include NGO fixed

Table 9-8. *Regressions of Results (Standard Errors)*

Indicator	Pay for performance	Constant	Number of observations	Number of groups	R^2
No contract period					
Full immunization	0.243***	0.672***	138	23	0.133
	(0.053)	(0.033)			
Three or more prenatal visits	0.109***	0.415***	151	26	0.052
	(0.042)	(0.025)			
Attended deliveries	0.269***	0.538***	126	24	0.087
	(0.057)	(0.036)			
Postnatal visits	0.099**	0.391***	126	26	0.024
	(0.05)	(0.031)			
Contract period					
Full immunization	0.132***	0.856***	138	23	0.315
	(0.053)	(0.049)			
Three or more prenatal visits	0.034	0.54**	151	26	0.09
	(0.045)	(0.042)			
Attended deliveries	0.196***	0.651***	126	24	0.087
	(0.61)	(0.056)			
Postnatal visits	0.023	0.51***	126	26	0.09
	(0.052)	(0.047)			

Source: Authors.
***$p < 0.01$
**$p < 0.05$

effects (table 9-8, rows 1 through 4) and contract period time effects (table 9-8, rows 5 through 9). Table 9-9 corresponds to table 9-8, except that the result attained is measured relative to the established target.

Results suggest that being paid based on performance is associated with a 13 to 24 percentage point increase in immunization coverage and a 17 to 27 percentage point increase in attended deliveries.

The effects are less consistent for prenatal and postnatal care. A highly significant 11 to 13 percentage point increase in prenatal care visits in the specification with NGO fixed effects is eroded when contract period effects are added. Postnatal care exhibits even weaker results that are further eroded when contract period effects are added. Possible explanations could be that returning for a minimum of three prenatal visits is determined less by the behavior of providers than by the action of patients. An additional challenge is that postnatal care was not included as an indicator in the first two contract periods.

Table 9-9. *Regressions of Difference between Results and Targets (Standard Errors)*

Indicator	Pay for performance	Constant	Number of observations	Number of groups	R^2
No contract period					
Full immunization	0.218***	−0.076**	125	23	0.120
	(0.052)	(0.032)			
Three or more prenatal visits	0.132**	−0.07***	169	26	0.035
	(0.033)	(0.034)			
Attended deliveries	0.218***	−0.073***	115	24	0.033
	(0.065)	(0.043)			
Postnatal visits	0.081	0.004	96	26	0.014
	(0.051)	(0.034)			
Contract period					
Full immunization	0.182***	−0.003***	125	23	0.179
	(0.056)	(0.051)			
Three or more prenatal visits	0.095	−0.005**	139	26	0.052
	(0.061)	(0.056)			
Attended deliveries	0.174***	0.008	115	24	0.047
	(0.69)	(0.063)			
Postnatal visits	0.07	0.21	96	26	0.026
	(0.057)	(0.049)			

Source: Authors.
***$p < 0.01$
**$p < 0.05$

Stakeholder Perceptions

Feedback from NGOs in 2005—Centres pour le Développement et la Santé, Comité Bienfaisance de Pignon, and the Haitian Health Foundation—strongly endorses performance-based payment (Bourdeau, Alfred, and Vincent 2005; Comité Bienfaisance de Pignon 2005; Despagne 2005).

—Pressure to achieve performance indicators resulted in strategies to motivate staff and fostered team spirit.

—Strong information systems developed to fulfill reporting requirements on health indicators resulted in the generation and use of reliable data.

—The burden of financial reporting was considerably reduced.

—Flexibility was gained in the use of funds.

—Valuable technical assistance became available, especially for self-assessment, program management, and supervision of family planning initiatives.

—The partners network contributed significantly to learning across organizations.
—The targets set were attainable and designed collaboratively.

Certain disadvantages were also mentioned, however, especially the institutional stress from the pressure to achieve results. NGOs pointed out that they sometimes had to work during bad weather and under challenging conditions to avoid losing the bonus. They expressed frustration at the all-or-nothing payment terms, which risked payment on an indicator that might be only a small fraction under the established target. They also noted that they were sometimes hindered by factors not under their control, citing their dependency on other institutions for certain commodities.

Project staff observed that although all NGOs receive a package of capacity-enhancing interventions, those participating in the performance-based payment scheme made more strategic choices in their technical assistance requests than their counterparts. Senior management in NGOs paid for results appear motivated to apply the adviser's recommendations rapidly. Specific areas of focus include the desire to strengthen information systems, stimulate staff interest in using program and financial information to make management decisions, and increase overall efficiency.

Another feature of the project that NGOs particularly valued was that they were frequently brought together as partners to share information, see how they performed relative to others, and learn from each other.

Conclusions

Paying for performance in Haiti is part of a package of interventions aimed at strengthening institutions to deliver quality health services to the Haitian population. Remarkable improvements in key health indicators have been achieved over the six years that payment for performance has been phased in. Now reaching 2.7 million people, NGOs in the project network provide essential services in the complicated context of violence, poverty, and limited government leadership.

This project offers a unique opportunity to examine trends over a period with progressively more NGOs graduating into performance-based payment. Performance on all indicators was stronger for the project as a whole than performance on similar indicators for the entire country. On average, performance-based NGOs in each contract period performed better than expenditure-based NGOs.

As with almost all evaluations of such programs, unambiguously concluding that performance-based payment is responsible for the results achieved or any portion of them is not possible. This is because other interventions were implemented simultaneously—such as technical assistance, opportunity to participate in a network and in cross-fertilization activities, and increased funding—making it hard to attribute improved performance to the incentive, to other interventions, or to a combination.

Evaluating NGO performance with self-reported data from NGOs, relying on audits to verify accuracy, is less expensive than contracting an independent firm to perform community and provider surveys. It also encourages NGOs to strengthen information systems and use information effectively to track performance and to know where to intervene. The impact of other design changes is less clear, however. The project made many changes in performance targets, moving from specified indicators to a combination of some fixed and some randomly selected indicators. But it is not possible to conclude from the data which approach to selecting indicators generated the largest improvement.

In addition to the recorded results, anecdotal evidence and results of recent field assessments suggest that performance-based payment has played an important catalytic role in the organizational development of the institutions involved. This is reflected in the changed behavior of managers and service providers at all levels, who are observed to be more proactive, innovative, and focused on being more accountable for results. These behavioral changes have resulted in improved information systems and the effective use of data for decision-making; strategic use of technical assistance; improvements in human capacity development and management (including training, decentralization, delegation, and supervision); stronger financial management; and increased cost-effectiveness. All of these changes will likely contribute to the long-term viability of these organizations.

Possible future enhancements of the project include introducing performance-based payments for the public sector and experimenting more with incentives tied to both HIV and tuberculosis care. Lessons will continue to be learned.

References

Bourdeau, Royneld, Casmir Alfred, and Jean Frenel Vincent. 2005. "Haitian Health Foundation Experience in PBF." Presentation to donors providing health sector support. Port-au-Prince, Haiti, May 16.

Collymore, Yvette. 2004. "Haiti's Health Indicators Reflect Its Political and Economic Pains." Washington: Population Reference Bureau. (www.prb.org [October 2008].)

Comité Bienfaisance de Pignon. 2005. "Experience en performance base." Presentation to donors providing health sector support. Port-au-Prince, Haiti, May 16.

Despagne, Pierre D. 2005. "Financement basé sur la performance: L'expérience des CDS." Presentation to donors providing health sector support. Port-au-Prince, Haiti, May 16.

Eichler, Rena. 2002. "Why Pay for Inputs When Better Health Comes from Paying for Results? Effective Steering through Strategic Purchasing Improves Health Indicators in Haiti." Washington: World Bank, Inter-American Development Bank, Pan American Health Organization, and International Graduate School of Management in Barcelona.

Eichler, Rena, Paul Auxila, and John Pollock. 2001. "Promoting Preventive Health Care: Paying for Performance in Haiti." In *Contracting for Public Services: Output-Based Aid and Its Applications,* edited by Penelope J. Brook and Suzanne Smith. Washington: World Bank.

PAHO (Pan American Health Organization). 2007. "The Challenge of Haiti." Washington. (www.paho.org/english/d/csu/TheChallengeofHaiti.pdf [October 2008].)

10

Rwanda: Performance-Based Financing in the Public Sector

Louis Rusa, Miriam Schneidman, Gyuri Fritsche, and Laurent Musango

---

Highlights

Countrywide implementation demonstrates that a national performance-based financing approach with both the public and private nonprofit health facilities is feasible in low-income countries.

Incentives reward both quantity and quality of curative, maternal and child health, and HIV/AIDS services.

Donor-funded pilots provided the evidence for the government of Rwanda to implement performance incentives as well as a menu of options that informed the design of a unified national model.

Rwanda is one of the pioneers of performance-based financing. Building on lessons from three donor-financed pilots, the government has assumed leadership for this approach and is scaling up a standardized model nationwide.

The authors would like to express appreciation to the individuals and groups who pioneered this approach in Rwanda and shared generously their time, information, and ideas. They would particularly like to thank Claude Sekabaraga (Ministry of Health), Agnes Soucat (World Bank), Jean Pierre Kashala and Cedric Ndizeye (HealthNet/Butare), Christian Habineza, Antonio Lozito, and Etienne Sekaganda (CORDAID/Cyangugu), Werner Vandenbulcke (Belgian Technical Cooperation), Bruno Meessen (Institute of Tropical Medicine, Antwerp), and Robert Soeters (public health and financing specialist). Bruno Meessen also provided detailed comments and suggestions on earlier drafts.

Performance-based financing is one of several strategies introduced to strengthen what was considered, according to the 2000 *World Health Report* rankings, one of the weakest health care systems in the world.

Between 1994 and 1996, following the war and genocide, user fees were abolished and then, in 1998, reintroduced. Use of health services subsequently hit bottom. The traditional approach of funding inputs (such as equipment, training, and drugs) did not generate good results. Providers were paid according to civil service rates, and accountability mechanisms were either weak or non-existent. The need to motivate and empower providers to produce better outcomes was critical. The pay-for-performance approach—*approche contractuelle,* as it is called in Rwanda—provided such an opportunity by financing results rather than inputs.

Although the scope and scale of the initial pilots were relatively modest, they nonetheless provided important information about details of design and implementation that informed the national scale-up. Participating health facilities received financial payments for incremental increases in the quantity of basic health services provided, such as immunization, prenatal care, and assisted deliveries. The overriding goal was to improve the use of health services by motivating providers. The goal of improving the quality of care was introduced more systematically only later. These schemes were applied to both public and private nonprofit health facilities administered by religious groups.

Based on lessons from these initial pilots, the government adopted a performance-based approach as a national policy in 2005. Its scale-up plan to reach national coverage was promptly launched, with a targeted completion date of May 2008. Mechanisms and instruments for the scale-up were put in place, along with an impact evaluation to strengthen the base of evidence for the approach.

At the same time, other health policy reforms were also being implemented to increase the use of key services by reducing demand-side barriers. To improve maternal health, women who participate in regular antenatal clinics receive free institutional deliveries. To protect against the financial risk imposed by health expenses and to encourage routine use of health services, community-based health insurance schemes (*mutuelles*) have been scaled up nationwide. This risk-pooling mechanism has contributed to higher use of primary health services for the insured and facilitated access to health services for the poor by subsidizing the premiums of needy households. At the same time, these demand-side interventions make it difficult to untangle the effects of the performance-based schemes that are aimed at motivating providers. However, evidence from the schemes does suggest that the performance-based approach offers the opportunity to achieve substantial results quickly in the delivery of health services, although the data reported do not control for the impact of demand-side policy interventions. A further potential bias could lie with the Imihigo performance contracts, between the president of the republic and mayors, which started in 2006 and include indicators related to the delivery of key services (for example, family planning, institutional deliveries, and access to community insurance schemes).

The Rwanda experience is unique because it represents a bold attempt to institutionalize an innovative approach, involves incentive payments for both basic health and communicable diseases, and entails a rigorous evaluation of impact.

Background

Rwanda is among the poorest countries in the world—the average Rwandan lives on less than $0.70 per day (U.S. dollars)—with a typical epidemiological profile for Sub-Saharan Africa. Although the genocide and war had a detrimental impact on health indicators, Rwanda is now slowly getting back on track in terms of the Millennium Development Goals, with good progress on lowering infant and under-five mortality. Nevertheless, malnutrition remains serious (45 percent of children under five are chronically malnourished), fertility rates are high (the total fertility rate is 6.1 percent), and maternal mortality is about 750 deaths per 100,000 live births (Haub 2006). The HIV adult prevalence rate is about 3 percent overall and 3.6 percent for women.

Per capita annual total health spending averages about $34, with donors funding more than 40 percent, government funding about one-third, and beneficiaries funding roughly one-quarter (World Health Organization 2003). In recent years, coverage with cost-effective interventions has improved somewhat. Coverage, however, remains generally inadequate, with large gaps between the poor and the nonpoor. The country has seen a rapid expansion in access to community health insurance, with government and donors subsidizing access to the poorest 25 percent of Rwandans in an effort to reduce inequities in access and health outcomes.

The 1994 genocide and war resulted in a massive loss of health professionals, destruction of health infrastructure, and general impoverishment of the population. In its immediate aftermath, Rwanda benefited from a substantial amount of external assistance that was used primarily to rebuild the country's physical infrastructure. By early 2000, donor support started to decline, and focus shifted from reconstruction to development assistance. The majority of health facilities in the country historically relied on revenues from user fees to finance their activities. The reintroduction of fees, following their abolishment after the genocide, imposed a burden on the population, and the country experienced a dramatic drop in the use of health services.

Exacerbating demand-side barriers to accessing care were weak incentives for service providers to reach the population. Salaries were fixed and very low and had no links to performance. To encourage health workers to serve in remote areas, some employees did receive salary top-ups, but they were not linked to performance. There were differences in pay and working conditions between the public and nonprofit sectors, causing physicians who were in short supply to migrate to the nonprofit sector, where salaries were somewhat higher. Salaries for other personnel were similar to what was offered in the public sector, but religious groups appeared to retain staff more effectively by inspiring loyalty or providing access to particular financial incentives, such as access to interest-free loans. Further perverse effects were created through funding based on inputs that resulted in greater resources for facilities with more staff, irrespective of performance.

The initial pay-for-performance schemes in the former provinces of Cyangugu and Butare were designed in this postconflict environment, which was characterized by low use, poor coverage, and inadequate incentives. Their main goal was to increase use by modifying the behavior of health providers through payment of incentives for a set of predetermined services.

Several factors facilitated the start-up in the pilot provinces of Cyangugu and Butare:

—Upgraded infrastructure with needed inputs: a well-established network of recently upgraded facilities regularly supplied with drugs,

—Physical access to services: 60 percent of the population within a 5-kilometer radius of a health center,

—Functioning public-private partnership: a functioning, historical partnership between government and nonprofit private facilities, which managed 60 and 40 percent, respectively, of all health facilities, and

—An adequate health information system, which is computerized and up-to-date.

The scale-up to the national level was made possible by Rwanda's commitment to good governance, essential to the performance-based approach, as evidenced by policies aimed at increasing accountability and enhancing the effectiveness of service delivery, such as the streamlining of central public sector ministries.

Prudent macroeconomic and fiscal management (reflected in annual gross domestic product growth of 7.4 percent between 1995 and 2005) enabled the government to increase priority spending in the social sectors. Health expenditures as a share of total government spending rose from 2.5 percent in 1998 to 11 percent in 2006.

Rwanda's track record of responsible and transparent use of donor funds also facilitated the adoption of the performance-based approach. For example, results from the World Bank HIV/AIDS project and from the Global Fund to Fight AIDS, Tuberculosis, and Malaria grants for HIV/AIDS have been strong, with all targets met and some exceeded. Budget support by the World Bank, European Commission, African Development Bank, United Kingdom, and Sweden have expanded rapidly, reflecting the confidence of donors in the management of funds.

Three Financing Schemes

The first two schemes were launched in 2002 by Dutch nongovernmental organizations (NGOs), one in Butare (Initiative pour la Performance) by HealthNet TPO and the other in Cyangugu by Memisa/CORDAID. The third project was undertaken in Kigali-Ngali, Kabgayi, and Kigali Ville in 2005 by Belgian Technical Cooperation (BTC), a development cooperation agency. The design of the first two was inspired by early lessons from a contracting initiative in Cambodia. The population covered by each scheme and the number of facilities involved at the time of start-up are presented in table 10-1.

The overriding goal of all three schemes was to increase the use of health services. This would be achieved by remunerating staff based partly on services delivered and by empowering them to identify creative ways to increase the quantity of those services. Expected innovations included subcontracting community groups and private dispensaries, introducing organizational changes, and recruiting

Table 10-1. *Population and Number of Facilities under Different Schemes at Start-up in Rwanda*

Location and time period	Population (millions)	Health centers	Hospitals	Health teams
Butare (2002)	0.4	36	3	4
Cyangugu (2002)	0.6	26	4	4
Kigali-Ngali, Kabgayi, Kigali Ville (2005)	1.6	75	4	4
Rwanda (2008, envisaged)	8.6	365	35	35

Source: Authors.

additional staff. The performance-based financing schemes were also expected to stimulate more effective management of facilities because providers had greater autonomy to decide how services would be organized and delivered. The common elements of and differences in the three schemes are included in appendix 10-1 and summarized here.

All schemes established clear management structures to institute payment agreements and pay facilities. In Cyangugu, the fund-holding international NGO was responsible for negotiating contracts, establishing fees, and making payments. In the BTC scheme, the bilateral donor comanaged the program with the Ministry of Health, working through the government structures. The Butare scheme went a step further in working with the provincial structures by creating a steering committee comprising the donor HealthNet TPO, the Ministry of Health, and the provincial health authorities. This committee negotiated a purchase contract with the health centers, which drew up motivation contracts for each employee (Meessen and others 2006).

Strategic planning was an integral aspect of the Butare and Cyangugu schemes. Health providers were required to prepare business plans in Cyangugu and encouraged to do so in Butare, with details on strategies for attaining results. At well-functioning facilities, the process of developing these plans was highly participatory and empowered stakeholders to find innovative ways to improve service delivery. Although the BTC scheme also involved staff in setting targets and identifying innovative approaches, strategic planning was not a key aspect.

The range of services was broadly similar. The goal of all three schemes was to cover progressively services in the basic health package for health centers and district hospitals. In Butare, the initial goal was to fund a set of "high-impact activities that were easy to deliver and easy to measure" (Meessen and others 2006). Services between 2002 and 2004 were thus provided at only the health facility level and in only two districts, both due to funding constraints and the desire to test the approach before embarking on the complexities of contracting hospitals. The Cyangugu scheme was relatively well financed and covered all facilities in the province, providing a more generous set of services, including payments for tuberculosis (TB) management, referrals, and obstetrical emergencies. The Butare and Cyangugu schemes introduced payments for HIV/AIDS services in mid-2005, and the BTC scheme did so for TB and malaria services.

The level of resources available varied across the schemes. The average per capita annual subsidy for each scheme depended on the services provided, resources available, and population served. This annual budget was about $0.24 per inhabitant per year in the Butare scheme, less than $0.20 in the BTC scheme, and about $2.00

in Cyangugu. The payments to facilities were made on a case-based reimbursement basis, with each additional output receiving a payment to reflect the incremental effort of staff. In Cyangugu, there was also an isolation bonus payment to assist facilities in geographically disadvantaged areas. The method of handling these payments also differed across the schemes. In Butare, where health centers had to inform the steering committee in advance of the pay scale for bonus payments, the money was given to the health committee, which then paid the staff. Some opted for retaining 5 percent for reinvesting at the facility level. In Cyangugu, payments were made directly to the facility, with health committees or management deciding how to use funds; on average, roughly 40 percent was given as staff bonus payments and 60 percent was reinvested at the facility. In the BTC scheme, facilities received payments and distributed them among personnel according to previously agreed criteria that captured the relative contributions of staff. On average, each health worker could earn between $25 and $30 monthly in the Butare and Cyangugu schemes before HIV performance bonus payments were introduced and around $18 in the BTC scheme, in addition to a predictable salary payment.

Each scheme used a different approach to monitor results and validate data. Each approach had its strengths and limitations. In Butare, the steering committee monitored results, limiting the need for additional personnel and funds. The scheme relied primarily on data generated by the Health Management Information System (HMIS), with periodic, random cross-checks. This obviated the need for a parallel information system, but did not always guarantee the reliability of data. However, according to key informants, one of the positive spillover effects was improved timeliness and accuracy of reporting. The Butare model also introduced third-party monitoring by commissioning the School of Public Health to survey client satisfaction every six months, but these surveys proved costly and infrequent. The Cyangugu scheme had a sophisticated and independent verification system, with supervisors and an officer for monitoring and evaluation to validate data and survey patient satisfaction. Having dedicated staff for monitoring acknowledges the importance of this function and highlights the need to earmark funds for this activity. The Cyangugu scheme also piloted an innovative civil society mechanism for monitoring results whereby community organizations conducted patient satisfaction surveys on a quarterly basis. Community representatives were chosen by the local community and included clergy, local leaders, wise men (*inyagamugayo*), and representatives of associations of people living with HIV/AIDS. Results of civil society monitoring were shared with facilities, which could receive a special award of a maximum of 15 percent on top of their monthly fees if their performance was deemed exceptional. The BTC scheme differed from the others by consolidating both supervision and data validation into one function, leading to much debate about a possible conflict of interest. But BTC administrators have argued that supervisors are remunerated on how well they perform their job (regularity of visits, timeliness of supervisory reports, and adequacy of follow-up measures) and not on how well the facilities under their supervision are performing.

The three pilot projects differed in the way quality of care was treated. In the Butare scheme, quality of care was not included, as it was considered complex to define and measure. In the Cyangugu scheme, district hospitals carried out a quality regulation function and awarded additional bonuses based on results. The BTC scheme developed a set of composite indicators as proxies for quality of care. At health centers, quality was defined in terms of adherence to protocols. At the hospital level, quality was assessed in terms of process indicators (such as timeliness of reports, lack of stock outs, and frequency of supervisory visits).

Results

Results from the three initial performance-based schemes show improvements in coverage, quality, and impact on patients. Nevertheless, the data need to be interpreted carefully for the following reasons:

—Analysis is limited to before and after observations and to comparison with noncontracting provinces.

—It is not possible to tease out the impact of other factors, such as the expansion in *mutuelle* coverage, that may also contribute to increasing use.

—Data are sometimes drawn from a relatively small sample of facilities and providers and cannot be viewed as representative or statistically significant.

—Information for all indicators was not available long enough to ascertain trends.

Cyangugu and Butare Schemes

The main source of comparative data is a World Bank–funded review that compared Butare and Cyangugu schemes with two provinces (Gikongoro, Kibungo) that benefited from substantial assistance but did not use the performance-based financing (PBF) approach. Data come from a combination of service statistics reported through the HMIS, surveys of a small sample of providers, and examination of quality in a sample of facilities. Quality was examined by randomly selecting eight health centers in the PBF regions of Cyangugu and Butare and comparing quality in eight randomly selected health centers from non-PBF regions of Gikongoro and Kibungo. These sixteen centers were surveyed by a team of one

Table 10-2. *Comparison of Services before and after the Intervention in Rwanda*

Province and time period	Curative care	Deliveries	Family planning	Measles
PBF provinces				
Before (2001)	0.22	12.2	1.1	70.7
After (2004)	0.55	23.1	3.9	81.5
Non-PBF provinces				
Before (2001)	0.20	6.7	0.3	77.9
After (2004)	0.30	9.7	0.5	78.9

Source: Authors.

supervisor from Cyangugu and an independent former supervisor from Butare. This team verified data and assessed quality by examining a small sample of patient files in each health center to determine appropriateness of care. Each health center could score one point for each of thirteen indicators of quality, and each province could score a maximum of fifty-two points (four health centers times thirteen points). Although it is difficult to attribute the improvements only to the performance-based approach, it is worth noting that others have found similar results when comparing PBF and non-PBF provinces in Rwanda, with findings from the Butare and Cyangugu schemes published in international peer-reviewed literature.

Coverage

Provinces with performance-based financing reported the largest increases in the quantities of both curative and preventive care services. Starting from a low of about 0.2 curative care visit per person per year in all provinces, performance-based financing provinces reached 0.5 visit per person per year, and non–performance-based provinces provided only 0.3 curative care visit per person per year. Between 2001 and 2004, the PBF group saw an increase of institutional deliveries of close to 11 percentage points, while the non-PBF group increased by only 3.0 percentage points (see table 10-2). Butare more than tripled coverage compared to Gikongoro (see figure 10-1). According to key informants, the boost in institutional deliveries was primarily due to innovative strategies to attract women to deliver at health centers, such as the establishment of additional centers to bring services closer to beneficiaries, paying traditional birth attendants to bring women to health centers, and providing clothing for newborns as an incentive to attract women to deliver. On family planning acceptors, even though the absolute numbers remain low, the PBF group showed an increase of 2.8 percentage points compared to only

Figure 10-1. *Institutional Deliveries and Measles Coverage in Rwanda, 2001–04*

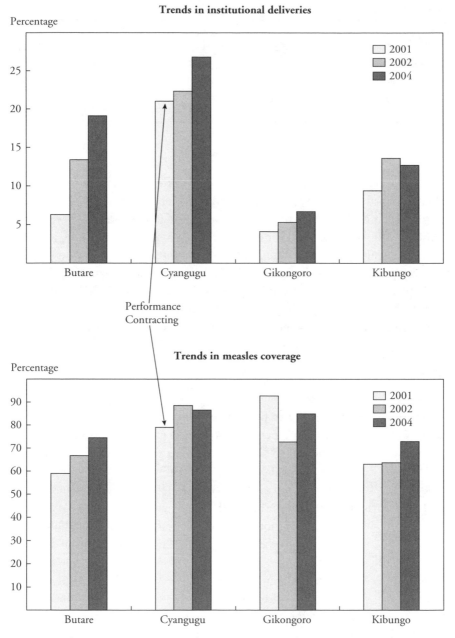

Source: Authors.

0.2 percentage point in the non-PBF group. On immunization, measles coverage increased by almost 11 percentage points in the PBF group, compared to only 1 percentage point in the non-PBF group. By 2004, the performance-based provinces slightly surpassed measles coverage in the non-performance-based provinces.

Quality

Performance-based provinces outperformed non-performance-based ones with a composite quality score of 73 versus 47 percent. Scores were considerably higher for effective management of deliveries and referral systems, but identical for other services, such as immunization. Provider satisfaction with income levels was relatively high in the contracting provinces, where staff received bonus payments of 27 percent (Butare) to 43 percent (Cyangugu) over and above their regular salaries. Views with respect to supervision were relatively positive in the contracting provinces, where roughly 80 percent of staff reported external supervision as frequent with effective follow-up; by contrast, only 44 percent of respondents in non-contracting provinces responded favorably. Virtually all staff involved in the contractual approach felt that it contributed to improved motivation, and about half mentioned qualitative improvements as a benefit.

In regard to impact on patients, although overall financing went up across the board, it increased at a faster rate in the contracting provinces, with a commensurate drop in out-of-pocket expenditures. Consumers paid less out of pocket in Butare and Cyangugu than in the noncontracting provinces. Consumers also accounted for about 85 percent of total spending in 2002 in all provinces, 68 percent in noncontracting provinces, but only about 51 percent in the contracting provinces.

BTC Scheme

At the time this chapter was written, information on the BTC scheme was available only for the period between 2004 and 2005; in spite of the short duration, it suggests several interesting results and early lessons (see table 10-3). The performance-based approach can generate results in a relatively limited timeframe. Progress has been made on most priority services (except prenatal care), with the BTC scheme reaching roughly 2 million inhabitants. Although it is not possible to attribute these improvements to the performance-based scheme alone, key stakeholders believe that the scheme has contributed greatly by establishing a results-oriented culture, strengthening supervision, and promoting innovative strategies for improving coverage.

Table 10-3. *Impact on Core Services in BTC Scheme in Rwanda, 2004 and 2005*
Proportion of target population served

Core service	2004	2005
Curative consultation	47.6	57.3
Prenatal consultation	53.2	52.2
Family planning	10.6	15.7
Growth monitoring	46.5	93.6
Immunization	80.0	83.6
Assisted deliveries	21.2	29.7
Treatment of severe malnutrition of children under five	1.5	4.0

Source: Authors.

Institutional deliveries increased, in part because of important innovations supported by the performance-based scheme. Other policies, such as the expansion in *mutuelles,* may also have influenced the positive trend in institutional deliveries, but the introduction of bonus payments for women who spend three days after delivery at a health center was an innovation of the contracted providers. Figure 10-2 shows an increase of more than 65 percent within nine months among such women. A sustained rise in institutional deliveries, combined with the three-day stay, may have an important impact on reducing complications from childbirth because it allows providers to identify immediate complications or problems with the newborns.

Improvement in curative consultations may be attributed only partly to the performance-based scheme. Program administrators believe that curative consultations are more sensitive to membership in *mutuelles* because members tend to use health facilities more often than nonmembers.

HIV/AIDS

Taking advantage of the existence of the performance-based schemes in Butare and Cyangugu, a core group of HIV/AIDS indicators was introduced in 2005 in the context of the World Bank–funded HIV/AIDS Multi-Sectoral Project. The performance-based approach was seen as a way to motivate staff to scale up HIV/AIDS services quickly. However, immediately after the introduction of the HIV/AIDS indicators, facilities noted that the bonus payments did not address the critical shortage of human resources, which prevented them from scaling up. Hence, in addition to the bonus payments, each district hospital received an annual grant of about $60,000. Hospitals had full authority to determine

Figure 10-2. *Institutional Deliveries in Rwanda, 2005 and 2006*

Number of deliveries

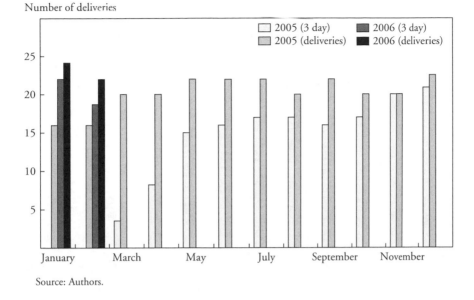

Source: Authors.

the number, profile, and payment levels of the additional personnel recruited. The Bank project used a learn-by-doing approach, which subsequently informed the financing of HIV/AIDS bonus payments by the President's Emergency Plan for AIDS Relief (PEPFAR) and the Global Fund to Fight AIDS, Tuberculosis, and Malaria.

A rapid scale-up of key HIV/AIDS services occurred after the introduction of the scheme, particularly in Cyangugu (see figure 10-3). Although the usual caveats apply in any before-and-after comparison, such as the lack of control groups and potential pilot-test bias, it is likely that the performance-based approach contributed to the increase in HIV testing and to the increase in couple testing, particularly as facilities used innovative strategies to reach more people. Within the first year, Cyangugu had surpassed the targets set under the World Bank operation and experienced an overall fourfold increase in monthly testing.

By contrast, there was no clear trend in the number of people on antiretroviral treatment at sites with and without the approach, even though sites with the approach appear to be doing slightly better (see figure 10-4). Before-and-after comparisons are influenced by several other factors, such as initial waiting lists, capacity to conduct CD4 counts, and decentralization of care to health centers,

Figure 10-3. *HIV Monthly Tests before and after Introduction of the PBF Scheme in Two Provinces of Rwanda*[a]

Percentage

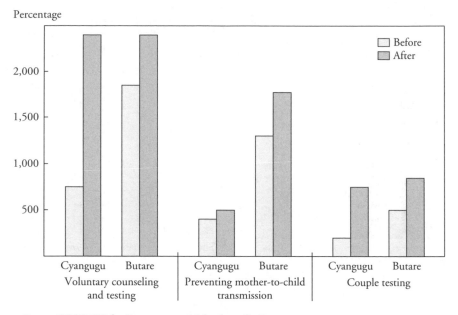

Cyangugu   Butare | Cyangugu   Butare | Cyangugu   Butare
Voluntary counseling and testing | Preventing mother-to-child transmission | Couple testing

Source: CORDAID for Cyangugu; *comité de pilotage* for Butare.
a. For Cyangugu before-after estimates refer to 2004 versus 2005–06; for Butare before-after estimates refer to 2005 versus 2006.

with patients assigned for follow-up to health centers. Focus group discussions with key informants suggested that the annual grants provided to hospitals were one of the key factors influencing the scale-up of services.

The introduction of HIV indicators in the performance-based schemes boosted staff salaries and may have contributed to the overall strengthening of the health system. The fee structure for HIV indicators under the two schemes was identical. But proportionately revenues from HIV represented a much larger share of total revenues under the Butare scheme because financing for basic health was relatively modest. As a result, a nurse working at a facility in Butare with the performance-based scheme earned, on average, about $80 monthly in comparison to roughly $30 for a nurse working at a nonparticipating health center. This distortion is gradually being phased out because virtually all facilities will shortly be participating in the PBF approach. Concerns were also raised by some stakeholders about the potential perverse effects of these funds resulting in the neglect of non-

Figure 10-4. *Monthly Uptake of Patients Receiving Antiretroviral Treatment before and after Introduction of the PBF Scheme in Rwanda*[a]

Number of patients receiving treatment

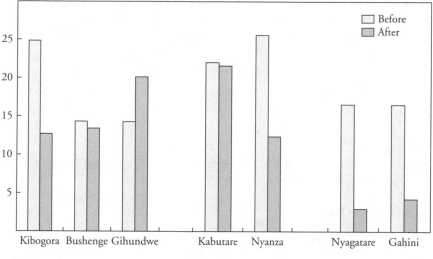

Source: Author.
a. Nyagatare and Gahini are comparison areas without performance-based financing.

HIV/AIDS patients. Program managers noted that there was no decline in other services in the same period and that facilities appeared to act rationally by using the infusion of additional HIV/AIDS resources to reinvest in facilities.

Scale-Up

Encouraging results from three pilots prompted the Ministry of Health to scale up a national model of performance-based financing. Key functions remain within the public system, with broad-based participation of providers, civil society, and local government. The scale-up began with three key actions: putting in place the institutional framework, standardizing the performance-based approach and tools, and developing a rollout plan and an impact evaluation.

Institutional Framework

Performance-based financing was adopted as a national policy as part of the 2005–09 Health Strategic Plan and subsequently incorporated into the National

Finance Law. The government developed specific statutes affecting health professionals that covered bonus payments to staff at both public and nonprofit health centers and district hospitals. In the short term, the government assumed responsibility for financing payments of about $0.25 per capita at all health centers, but urged development partners to continue temporarily funding district hospitals.

A thematic group on the performance-based approach was established to bring stakeholders together to exchange information and experiences. Key development partners—Belgium, the United States (PEPFAR), and the World Bank through the Poverty Reduction Support Credit/Grants[1]—have been instrumental in supporting the scale-up. The World Bank has spearheaded the design and rollout of the impact evaluation. CORDAID, HealthNet TPO, and BTC—the partners who supported the initial performance-based schemes—have been mobilized to assist in the scale-up, with technical support from the United States through Management Sciences for Health.

Approach and Tools

Based on the experience of the initial schemes, a standardized set of core services, a unique fee structure, and contracts were developed. The national plan involves delivery of core services at health centers and a complementary group of HIV/AIDS and hospital services. At the community level, a package of services and information will be provided.

Under the PBF scheme, health centers are reimbursed for the quantity of services provided according to a standardized fee structure for a list of fourteen services, adjusted by a composite quality score. Health centers can raise revenues by increasing the quantity of these services delivered and by improving quality. Bonus payments to health centers are calculated as follows:

$$\text{Health center PBF earnings} = (\text{fees} * \text{quantity}) * (\% \text{ quality score}).$$

Other sources of health center revenue are derived from government funding of health workers, user fees, *mutuelle* membership fees, and donor contributions. Quality is assessed quarterly by a team from the district hospital using a supervisory check list that measures thirteen services and 185 variables. A score of 100 percent

---

1. The World Bank–funded Poverty Reduction Support Credit/Grants have supported the performance-based financing and budgeting for service delivery with the goal of reaching the Millennium Development Goals. They have been funded jointly with the African Development Bank Group, the International Monetary Fund, the U.K. Department for International Development, Germany, the Netherlands, and Sweden.

would provide health centers with their full payment. Scores of less than 100 percent discount the payment proportionately.

Hospital budgets are determined prospectively, based on an annual value of about $600 per bed. Each quarter, quality is assessed through a peer review system (a team from a peer hospital assesses the quality of another similar hospital). Hospitals are provided points for achievements along a checklist of fifty-one composite indicators organized into three main categories: administration, quality assurance, and clinical activities. All hospitals have a specific point value (as determined by their individual prospective global budgets), and 100 percent performance is equivalent to the maximum number of points that can be gained. Roughly 50 percent of the budget is allocated for outputs, 30 percent for quality, and 20 percent for administration. Most hospitals, one year into the hospital PBF model, score around 80 percent each quarter. In addition, hospitals that offer HIV/AIDS services have the opportunity to earn additional revenues by providing HIV/AIDS services included on a specified list. These added revenues are calculated by multiplying the quantity of each service on a list by the assigned fee, discounted by the quality score assigned to the hospital in that quarter.

District steering committees negotiate three types of performance contracts: those between the Ministry of Health and the thirty administrative districts, performance contracts between district steering committees and the health center management committees, and motivation contracts between the health center committees and individual health workers.

For data verification and validation, the scale-up plan drew on the most promising aspects of the earlier schemes. Data entry and retrieval are performed through the Internet. District PBF steering committees validate invoices quarterly. Data are validated by specially trained data agents from the district health department (under the Ministry of Local Administration) or from a specially designated team from the district hospital. The district hospital team checks quality on a quarterly basis. The PBF steering committees validate bills and send them to the Ministry of Health to approve quarterly district payments, through the Ministry of Finance, into health center bank accounts. Both government and other purchasers use the same health facility bank accounts to transfer quarterly payments. Rwanda's relatively well-performing public finance system facilitates this simple flow of funds, which augurs well for the national scale-up. A multistage random sampling of both quantity data, which will use client satisfaction surveys in the community, and quality data, which will revalidate randomly sampled quality checklists, are planned for 2008.

Table 10-4. *Impact Evaluation Timeline in Rwanda*

	Implementation		Impact evaluation
Time period	Phase 1	Phase 2	surveys
2006			
January			Baseline, general health
March			
June–September	Start intervention		Baseline, HIV/AIDS
2007			
2008			
February–April			Follow-up
April		Start intervention	

Source: Authors.

Impact Evaluation

Despite promising results from the performance-based schemes, it was widely agreed that a rigorous impact evaluation was needed to inform public policy. An evaluation scheme was thus initiated to assess the impact on health status and on service delivery in terms of quantity, quality, and provider motivation. A rollout plan was developed, with districts matched on key characteristics and grouped into treatment and control groups. Thirteen districts covered by the initial schemes continue the performance-based approach, adopting the national PBF model, ten districts started in 2006 (phase one), and the remaining seven serve as control groups, introducing the scheme in April and May 2008 (phase two). The impact evaluation strategy was to measure the health situation before the start of the package, in both phase one and phase two areas (the baseline), and to measure the health situation again before the start of the package in the phase two areas (the follow-up survey). In order not to hinder the scale-up of key programs and to avoid creating large inequities between participating and nonparticipating districts, phase two districts received a lump-sum payment, equivalent to the average quarterly earnings of phase zero and one health facilities, but they did not participate in the performance-based scheme. The evaluation strategy uses the rollout plan for the national scale-up (see table 10-4).

Conclusions

The Rwanda experience has shown that performance-based schemes can generate rapid results on a large scale in terms of expanding use and coverage, particularly for services that are easy to deliver and measure. This finding is similar to that found in other developing-country settings. The performance-based approach in Rwanda engendered a results-oriented culture that promoted managerial autonomy and empowered providers to find creative solutions, such as subcontracting birth attendants and establishing new health posts. It also created an environment in which the government has gained enough confidence to decentralize the recruitment and dismissal of health professionals to health centers and hospitals. Most important, it has demonstrated that providers know their local conditions and have the skills and knowledge to deliver desired results. Furthermore, the performance-based schemes have contributed to strengthening normative functions through enhanced monitoring, planning, and supervision. Contracts that stipulate deliverables strengthen accountability at all levels.

Performance-based schemes are neither a panacea for all problems of health systems nor a substitute for investments in health facilities. They are just one promising and innovative strategy to tackle issues related to service use and provider performance. The Rwanda experience has shown that they can work in a resource-constrained environment, but only when minimal conditions are in place, such as a functioning drug supply system, minimal staffing levels, and the autonomy to recruit and dismiss personnel.

The jury is still out on whether financial incentives are the key motivating factor behind the boost in health sector performance in Rwanda. Key informants and program managers differ on the relative importance of the payments and the empowering effect of the approach. Some stakeholders believe that financial payments made a significant difference in a context where salaries remain inadequate. Others argue that the intrinsic nature of the performance-based approach is what mattered most. In the words of one key informant, the performance-based approach helped to generate team spirit. Clearly, financial payments that boosted salaries by more than 40 percent had a large motivational impact, as reflected in the greater reported satisfaction with working conditions in Cyangugu. But even in cases where payments were relatively modest, as in Butare, important increases in service delivery were registered. Another important factor is the enhanced supervision by district health teams, an integral part of the approach. Key informants reported a discernible improvement in the supervisory function in all areas where the schemes were introduced. This is consistent with findings from other settings, where enhanced supervision itself proved a powerful factor for change in public health systems.

The pilot phase generated important lessons for the national scale-up. First, determining the optimal fund-holding arrangement for the contracting scheme needs to balance capacity concerns with government ownership. Although in two of the initial schemes the funds were held by an NGO or bilateral agency with strong technical capacity, for the national scale-up the government opted to retain this function in the public system, but with strong civil society representation. Rwandan authorities felt that this was important to ensure that the fund holder was accountable to the government, rather than to the donors, and that institutional capacity for contract management was put in place in the public system.

Second, the quality dimension is critical and needs to be built into the design of these schemes. Although the initial focus in the immediate postconflict period was on increasing the use of services, quality dimensions were subsequently incorporated into the national model, with a mechanism to adjust payments for quality of care. This approach introduces incentives to maintain and improve quality. Nevertheless, as in other countries, there remain enormous challenges to defining and measuring quality, and the process should be flexible, using a learn-by-doing approach.

Third, putting in place an efficient and cost-effective system to validate the accuracy of data and monitor patient satisfaction is essential to the success of this approach. As in other settings, the Rwanda experience has confirmed that the process of verifying the accuracy of data should not be overly onerous or costly. Indicators should be easy to verify, the number of indicators should be kept reasonable, and the quality of care should be verified only periodically. The use of community associations in the Cyangugu scheme proved a promising and innovative way to empower civil society groups in this process.

Finally, indicators need to be reviewed and revised in a learn-by-doing environment to ensure that they are clearly articulated and provide the right incentives. Close consultation with end users of both quality and quantity indicators at the health center and hospital levels is a good practice that ensures ownership by health facilities and district authorities.

The impact on patients appears generally positive, as the use of services rose and the quality of care appeared to improve. In Cyangugu, there was a concerted effort to entice health managers to lower out-of-pocket payments to reduce financial barriers and improve use. This was not the case in the other provinces, but it is a strategy some providers may select in the future. The impact on the poor remains unclear. On a general note, the services provided focus on the needs of the poor, and many of those served at contracting sites are poor. For the individuals who benefited from the expansion in health services, benefits were clear. For services that already had high coverage levels, the incremental benefits accrued to those hardest to reach. But, overall, the approach did not have the explicit objective of targeting the poor because this is being done primarily by paying premiums for poor households to access the *mutuelles*.

The performance-based approach runs the risk of exacerbating inequities among health providers, and thus mitigation measures need to be built into the schemes. Providers do not always compete on an equal footing. As in other countries, staffing levels vary among facilities, and some serve groups in remote areas. The use of an isolation bonus, as in Cyangugu, assisted facilities in such areas to compete to attract health workers.

One of the key concerns is whether and how the results achieved so rapidly can be sustained with the national scale-up. The good news is that the two initial schemes have had more than five years of sustained experience in providing a broad range of services and operating at a large number of facilities. That the government has now assumed financial responsibility for the bonus payments, initially at health centers, augurs well for financial sustainability by lowering the dependence on external funding. At the same time, successful performance-based schemes may attract other donors, such as the United States, which is now supporting the scheme, and the Global Fund to Fight AIDS, Tuberculosis, and Malaria, which will become an important contributor of HIV/AIDS performance-based financing payments starting in 2008. By the same token, however, institution building will need to keep pace with the government's ambitious rollout plan. Key stakeholders report tremendous enthusiasm among district authorities, but the task of putting in place capacities for contract management, data validation, and supervision at some 400 health centers nationwide should not be underestimated. Mobilizing experts continues to be pivotal in the rollout of the national program. Technical assistance needs to be sustained until the new system is up and fully running.

One of the single most important lessons emerging from early experience with the performance-based approach in Rwanda is the need for rigorous evaluation. Consensus among key stakeholders on the benefits of the approach and evidence suggests that it is promising, even though it has not always been possible to tease out the effects of other factors contributing to improvements in coverage or to ascertain the counterfactual. The proposed national scale-up offers the opportunity to test the approach under different conditions. The impact evaluation now under way is expected to provide important evidence for future policies.

Appendix 10-1. Key Features of Schemes

What is the population covered?

—Butare: Gakoma (about 304,400) and Kabutare (roughly 80,000) districts, with a total population of about 384,400.
    —Cyangugu: Roughly 640,000 inhabitants province-wide.
    —Kigali-Ngali: About 1.6 million in 2005.

When was the scheme initiated?

—Butare: The pilot phase was initiated in early 2002. The program started in March 2002 in Gakoma and in June 2002 in Kabutare, or roughly four years ago.
    —Cyangugu: The pilot project was initiated in June 2002 in two health districts and was scaled up to provincial level in January 2003 or about 3.5 years ago.
    —Kigali-Ngali: The pilot project in Rutongo health district was carried out during 2003–04. Scale-up was initiated in January and February 2005 or roughly 1.5 years ago.

Why was scheme introduced?

—Butare: The key motivation for the start-up of this scheme was the poor performance of the health system as measured by the decline in use of key health services. With the reintroduction of user fees after the war, patients spent on average for each episode about RF 437 in comparison to RF 175 a few years earlier.
    —Cyangugu: An evaluation carried out in 2002 found that results based on an input approach were not satisfactory. A household study (January 2003) identified problems of access and use. Provincial authorities decided to adopt an output-based approach province-wide. By January 2003 all twenty-four health centers and four district hospitals had signed contracts.
    —Kigali-Ngali: The scheme was introduced province-wide based on the initial positive results of the pilot project in the Rutongo health district.

Which facilities are covered?

—Butare: Initially only health centers were included in the performance scheme supported by Initiative pour la Performance, but the scheme was gradually expanded to include district hospitals.
    —Cyangugu: All twenty-four health centers and four district hospitals in public and NGO sectors and nineteen private dispensaries are covered.
    —Kigali-Ngali: All health centers and district hospitals in areas where the scheme operates are covered.

Who is the payer?

—Butare: The steering committee (*comité de pilotage*) makes payments.

—Cyangugu: An international NGO (CORDAID) mobilizes funds from different sources (for example, central government, province, and donors, including International Development Association, United Nations Population Fund, the Netherlands). The fund holder verifies that the data are correct.

—Kigali-Ngali: Belgian Technical Cooperation.

Do providers prepare strategic plans?

—Butare: Yes, the health center management committee (*comité de gestion*) has the responsibility to develop strategic plans. One of the main features of the Butare scheme was to encourage innovation in service delivery. The *comité de gestion* includes representatives of health centers and the population.

—Cyangugu: Yes, strategic plans are prepared on a quarterly and annual basis and are a condition for accessing funds

—Kigali-Ngali: Quantitative and qualitative targets are set in consultation between Belgian Technical Cooperation and providers. No strategic plans are produced.

What services are provided at the health facility level?

—Butare: Health centers provide curative consultations, prenatal visits, assisted and referred deliveries, immunization, family planning, TB services, voluntary counseling and testing (VCT), and preventing mother-to-child transmission (PMTCT) services. District hospitals provide consultations, hospitalization, surgeries, referred deliveries, obstetrical emergencies, vasectomies and ligatures, TB screening and diagnosis, intrauterine device and norplant insertions, documented deaths, and VCT, PMTCT services, and antiretroviral therapy.

—Cyangugu: Health centers provide curative consultations, prenatal visits, assisted deliveries, immunization, family planning, VCT, and PMTCT services. District hospitals provide consultations, hospitalization, surgeries, complex deliveries, vasectomies and ligatures, VCT, PMTCT services, and antiretroviral therapy.

—Kigali-Ngali: Minimum Package of Activities (health center), Curative Package of Activities (district hospital), and management activities.

What services are provided at the community level?

—Butare: Impregnated bed nets, diphtheria, pertussis, tetanus dropouts, and outreach.

—Cyangugu: Impregnated bed nets.

—Kigali-Ngali: Home visits and promotional activities by community health workers.

How are targets set?

—Butare: Targets are set by the health committee members.

—Cyangugu: Targets are set based on national objectives and translated into what is feasible locally (that is, health center catchment area).

—Kigali-Ngali: Quantitative targets are set taking into account international standards of optimal coverage and local conditions. Qualitative targets are instructions to be found in the diagnostic and treatment records specific for each type of activity.

What is the average per capita annual subsidy or premium payment?

—Butare: Roughly $0.30 equivalent.

—Cyangugu: About $2.00 equivalent.

—Kigali-Ngali: About $1.60 equivalent.

How much is staff receiving in terms of incremental payments?

—Butare: About $25 equivalent.

—Cyangugu: Between $25 and $30 equivalent.

—Kigali-Ngali: Up to $20 equivalent.

Who receives payments, and how are these funds used?

—Butare: Health centers receive payments based on the number of services provided monthly; the *contrat global d'achat* is between the health center and the *comité de pilotage;* funds are used for individual payments and vary according to the number of services provided. A second contract is established between the health center management committee and each individual staff member.

—Cyangugu: The subsidies are paid directly to the facility. The health facility committees decide on the use of funds; on average roughly 40 percent is given as a bonus to staff, and 60 percent is reinvested at the facility level.

—Kigali-Ngali: The facility receives the payments and distributes them among the personnel, taking into account their qualification and grade level.

Is supervision remunerated?

—Butare: No, district supervisors are not remunerated.

—Cyangugu: The district health team conducts supervision.

—Kigali-Ngali: Yes, district supervisors receive RF 40,000 ($73) monthly, assuming timely and correctly filled out monthly reports.

How are data validated?

—Butare: *Comité de pilotage* ensures that the contracts are well carried out and takes corrective measures if problems emerge.

—Cyangugu: The fund holder validates the quantitative data; the district team also monitors and assesses the quality of care using standardized national tools for basic health and for HIV/AIDS; the district teams can approve up to a 15 percent bonus payment for quality.

—Kigali-Ngali: Data on quantitative indicators in registers are verified directly, and the records used for each subsidized activity are counted using simple indicators of quality.

Are there periodic surveys to measure patient satisfaction or validate results?

—Butare: Yes, the School of Public Health carries out periodic surveys to validate the accuracy of data.

—Cyangugu: Local community groups or associations conduct patient satisfaction surveys on a quarterly basis, increasing the voice of consumers.

—Kigali-Ngali: No additional surveys are carried out.

References

Haub, Carl. 2006. *Rwanda Demographic and Health Survey 2005.* Washington: Population Reference Bureau. (www.prb.org/Articles/2006/RwandaDemographicandHealthSurvey2005.aspx [October 2008].)

Meessen, Bruno, Laurent Musango, Jean-Pierre Kashala, and J. Lemlin. 2006. "Reviewing Institutions of Rural Health Centers: The Performance Initiative in Butare, Rwanda." *Tropical Medicine and International Health* 11 (8): 1303–17.

WHO (World Health Organization). 2003. *Guide to Producing National Health Accounts.* Geneva. (www.who.int/nha/docs/English_PG.pdf [October 2008].)

Additional Readings

Kalk, Andreas, and others. 2005. "Paying for Health in Two Rwandan Provinces: Financial Flows and Flaws." *Tropical Medicine and International Health* 10 (9): 872–78.

Loevinsohn, Benjamin, Erlinda T. Guerrero, and Susan P. Gregorio. 1995. "Improving Primary Health Care through Systematic Supervision: A Controlled Field Trial." *Health Policy Plan* 10 (2): 144–53.

Loevinsohn, Benjamin, and April Harding. 2005. "Buying Results? Contracting for Health Service Delivery in Developing Countries." *Lancet* 366 (August): 676–81.

Meessen, Bruno, Jean-Pierre Kashala, and Laurent Musango. 2007. "Output-Based Payment to Boost Staff Productivity in Public Health Centers: Contracting in Kabutare District, Rwanda." *Bulletin of the World Health Organization* 85 (2): 85–160.

Meessen, Bruno, Laurent Musango, and Jean-Pierre Kashala. 2004. *L'initiative pour la performance.* Ministry of Health and HealthNet International, Kigali, Rwanda.

Musango, Laurent, Gyuri Fritsche, Cedric Ndizeye, Ousmane Faye, Apolline Uwayitu, Alex Hakuzimana, Kathy Kantengwa, and John Pollock. 2007. "Provider Payment Mechanisms Using Performance-Based Financing/Performance-Based Contracting, Report on Progress in the Rwanda PRSP from the Government of Rwanda." Ministry of Health.

Soeters, Robert, and Fred Griffiths. 2003. "Improving Government Health Services through Contract Management: A Case from Cambodia." *Health Policy and Planning* 18 (1): 74–83.

Soeters, Robert, Laurent Musango, and Bruno Meessen. 2005. *Comparison of Two Health OBA Schemes in Rwanda.* Washington: World Bank.

Soeters, Robert, Jean Perrot, Etienne Sekaganda, and Antonio Lozito. 2006. "Purchasing Health Packages for the Poor through Performance-Based Contracting: Which Changes in the District Health System Does It Require?" Paper presented at the second international conference Health Financing in Developing Countries. Centre de'Etudes et de Recherches sur le Développement, Clermont Ferrand, France, December 1–2, 2005.

11

Nicaragua: Combining Demand- and Supply-Side Incentives

Ferdinando Regalía and Leslie Castro

Highlights

A conditional cash transfer program should incorporate both demand-side and supply-side performance incentives.

Significant improvements are seen in immunizations, growth monitoring, and reductions in stunting.

Two-phase impact evaluation does not disentangle the individual impacts of demand-side and supply-side incentives, but its results suggest that a well-targeted strategy of supply-side performance incentives could, on its own, be enough to achieve and maintain high levels of health care service use among poor rural populations.

The Red de Protección Social (RPS) is one of the first conditional cash transfer (CCT) programs implemented in a low-income country. Modeled after the Mexican program Progresa (now called Oportunidades), Nicaragua's CCT program is designed to address both current and future poverty by making cash transfers to poor households in rural areas. The transfers are conditional on the children in these households attending school and making visits to preventive health care providers. Monitoring and enforcing compliance with these conditions make RPS a demand-side pay-for-performance scheme, which addresses financial constraints that prevent individuals from accessing basic education and health services. By targeting poor households, the program alleviates short-term poverty; by linking the transfers to investments in human capital, the program aims to reduce long-term poverty (Maluccio and Flores 2005).

Although demand-side incentives are a key element, RPS is unique in that it complements these with supply-side incentives through a performance-based scheme to improve the use and quality of preventive health services among the very poor. Since the program's earliest stages, the government of Nicaragua recognized the urgent need to strengthen the supply of specific health care interventions in program areas so that beneficiary households could comply with the program's conditions. Two key implementation decisions were taken:

—Recognizing the inability of the Ministry of Health to expand services quickly to residents in remote localities, the government, for the first time, outsourced these services to private providers and nongovernmental organizations (NGOs) through competitive bidding.

—Contracted providers were to be paid based on their achievement of measurable and predetermined targets, verified by independent sources. This performance-based system was aimed at providing incentives for health providers to develop efficient plans to expand coverage rapidly in underserved areas.

The combination of providing performance-based awards in the form of monetary transfers to households and setting up incentives for health providers to attain performance targets proved an effective strategy to increase access to and improve the quality of basic health services in RPS localities. The RPS was conceived as a two-phase program, to be implemented over a period of five years, starting in 2000. The first phase, supported by the Inter-American Development Bank (IDB) and executed by the Nicaraguan Emergency Social Investment Fund (ESIF), was supposed to last three years, with a budget of $11 million. In 2002, as a condition of the IDB loan and to assess whether the program needed any modifications before its expansion, the government solicited external evaluations of the first phase. The International Food Policy Research Institute (IFPRI) conducted a quantitative impact evaluation using a randomized locality-based design.

Based in part on positive findings from the various evaluations, the government and IDB agreed in late 2002 to expand the program for three years, with a budget of $22 million. Execution of the second phase was passed to the Ministry of the Family to institutionalize the program within a line ministry. The original RPS design was modified to include a broader array of preventive health care interventions, reduce the size of transfers, and strengthen targeting tools. IFPRI also conducted a quantitative impact evaluation, using a quasi-experimental design, alongside a qualitative evaluation of the program's second phase. The results of both evaluations are inconclusive on the relative contribution of supply-side and demand-side incentives. But they do imply that the combination can increase the use of health services among the poor and improve health outcomes significantly.

Constraints

A CCT program aims to ease the budget constraints or the income-related demand constraints that families face when securing health care or education for their children. Cash transfers help families to cover the private costs—both direct and opportunity—of sending children to school or bringing them for preventive health checkups. Increasing the supply of services alone may not help because demand can remain constrained for reasons such as the high cost of accessing services, an imperfect knowledge of the long-term benefits of investing in human capital such as health and education, an environment of increased risk that reduces the incentive to invest in human capital for the long term, and social exclusion.

Demand for preventive health care of a given quality is influenced by whether an individual appreciates its value and is willing and able to seek it, which in turn depends on the direct and opportunity costs of accessing services. Recognizing these tensions and introducing demand-side, performance-based interventions such as CCTs that try to align consumer objectives with social goals have the potential to support care-seeking behavior (Eichler 2006).

When the RPS was designed, the evidence for demand-side constraints was stronger for education than for health. According to the 1998 Living Standards Measurement Survey, 48 percent of extremely poor children in Nicaragua cited economic reasons for not attending school, and 6 percent said rural labor activities kept them away. IFPRI's baseline data, collected for the impact evaluation, showed that in RPS localities only 58.9 percent of extremely poor children ages seven to thirteen were in school. The same figure was 65.7 and 81.7 percent, respectively, among the poor and the nonpoor (IFPRI 2001). This evidence strongly suggested income-related, demand-side constraints without being necessarily conclusive.

The evidence of demand-side constraints on the use of health services was quite limited. The IFPRI baseline data showed that only 66 percent of extremely poor children younger than three had received a health checkup in the six months before the data were collected in RPS localities. This figure was 73 percent among poor and 78 percent among nonpoor children. Other indicators, such as the percentage of children monitored for growth and development, demonstrated a similar pattern.

However, locality-specific RPS surveys from before the program began confirmed that supply constraints were much more binding in health than in education services, in terms of both access and quality. More than a third of RPS resources were therefore earmarked to strengthen the supply of preventive health services, with education receiving a smaller share.

During the first twenty-four months of program execution, the greatest impacts on service use in both education and health were observed among very poor households (IFPRI 2003), suggesting that constraints in demand (scarce household resources) were more binding than constraints in supply. Once the RPS began, all residents had to comply with the same set of conditions to receive transfers, facing fairly uniform access to and quality of preventive health services (Maluccio, Murphy, and Regalía 2006).

During program preparation, not enough data were available to determine either the private costs faced by households in accessing health care and education or the optimal size of the transfer, especially in health. The program estimated the average size of the transfer by taking into consideration the consumption-poverty gap, which is the difference between extremely poor households' average consumption and the official extreme poverty line. During the program's first phase, the average transfer was about 21 percent of recipients' total annual household expenditures before implementation of the program. In the second phase, the value of the average transfer was reduced by about 30 percent.

Cash versus Conditional Cash

RPS households received transfers if they sent their children to school and took them for health checkups. Making transfers conditional was justifiable on three grounds. Parents might not value the returns from investing in their children's health and education, possibly due to a lack of information on future returns. Their investment decisions would be suboptimal, and conditioning the transfer might enhance welfare for both parents and children. Parents might reasonably assess and value such returns but simply prefer to spend their money on other things, in which case conditions would impose a welfare loss for parents and enhance children's welfare. Parents could always opt out of the program. Investments in health and education would have large externalities that families would not internalize. In this case, conditions would address market failures and help to capture cross-sector effects.

Whatever the rationale for conditions, if household budget constraints are the main reason for suboptimal investment in the health and education of children, income transfers alone can increase the use of these services (Schady and Araujo 2006). The marginal contribution of conditions should be assessed against the costs of ensuring compliance. The design of the RPS impact evaluation did not allow an assessment of the relative contributions of factors related to income (transfers) and price (conditions) on the final outcomes. However, RPS impacts on the use of health and education services were higher among the very poor (IFPRI 2003), which suggests that income factors might have played a critical role, perhaps greater than conditions.

Although the increased income may have alleviated demand constraints and thus enabled households to use more health and education services, enforced compliance of RPS conditions boosted collective action at the municipal level to demand better coverage of services from the government, leading to more responsive supply. This empowerment factor is an important feature of CCT programs. If supply is not stepped up in response to demand-side incentives, conditions can frustrate beneficiaries and lead to calls for easing the monitoring of their compliance with program requirements, thereby diluting the conditionality aspect of the transfers.

Health Interventions

At the end of the 1990s, Nicaragua had levels of infant mortality well above the Central American average, a high prevalence of infectious and parasitic diseases, and pervasive malnutrition. Infant mortality accounted for the majority of all premature deaths. Malnutrition was the main factor underlying more than half of under-five mortality and 20 percent of maternal deaths (World Bank 2001).

Before the RPS program started, 37.9 percent of children younger than five living in RPS program areas suffered from retarded growth (stunting) because of malnutrition or illness (IFPRI 2001). This figure was 1.6 times greater than the national prevalence of stunting for this age group for 1997 and 1998 and nearly twenty times greater than the statistically expected prevalence for healthy populations. In program areas, the poorest 20 percent of children showed the highest levels of stunting (Maluccio and Flores 2005).

Access to health care was (and still is) characterized by large and persistent differences between the poor and nonpoor in Nicaragua. Extremely poor children reported illness 50 percent more frequently than children who were not poor, who, in turn, used health services 50 percent more frequently when they were sick. To access health care, the extreme poor had to travel three times the distance and spend three times as much to reach health facilities as their nonpoor counterparts (World Bank 2001). Before the program started in 2000, only 40 percent of children ages twelve to twenty-three months in RPS areas had received up-to-date vaccinations (IFPRI 2001). According to the 1998 Demographic and Health Survey, the vaccination coverage in rural areas was 68 percent. Before the program started, just above 70 percent of children younger than three in RPS areas had received any medical checkup during the previous six months (Maluccio and Flores 2005). As mentioned, service use was lower among the poorest households.

Given this background, the RPS health interventions during the first phase concentrated on preventive health care services for children younger than six that included child growth and development monitoring, vaccinations, antiparasite medicines, and micronutrients. Preventive health care providers referred sick children to the closest health unit. RPS providers held health educational workshops every two months on topics like household sanitation, nutrition, and reproductive health.

Before the program, some RPS localities had no access to preventive health services. Others did, supposedly, but often the closest health post could be reached only after many hours of walking. The RPS program provided service locations within an hour's walk from beneficiary families. Its biggest impact on access, however, came in its second phase, when it entered the impervious terrain of the Atlantic coast. In places like Wiwili, a vast and sparsely populated municipality on the border with Honduras, there were only nine health centers, often accessible only by an expensive, eight-hour boat ride. These centers were typically staffed only by auxiliary nurses because both doctors and medicines were in short supply. Since 2004, however, 325 service locations have been established and are visited regularly by private health teams from the municipal center.

Mothers bring their children to the local service location to be seen by the private provider's health care team. Teams are made up of three members, each with his or her own responsibilities according to a set protocol: a doctor, a professional nurse, and an auxiliary nurse, psychologist, or nutritionist. Transporting vaccines to the most remote localities and preserving the integrity of the cold chain were a logistical challenge, which was often met with the support of the communities by placing, for example, refrigerators that run on gas in key locations.

During the RPS's second phase, the menu of health interventions was expanded to include sexual reproductive health, maternal health, and vaccination boosters for children between six and nine years old. *Promotoras*—beneficiary women selected by the community—were present when services were delivered and thus acquired training on the job. They became an important part of a network of human resources capable of the tasks associated with nutritional counseling and child growth monitoring.

Demand Side: Transfers

With limited information on national poverty rates, the RPS team had to determine the best way to identify the program's target population of extremely poor rural households with children under fourteen. During the first phase, the team wanted to compare the effectiveness of two targeting options: only geographic targeting and geographic combined with household-level targeting. They used geographic targeting to select departments, municipalities and, within municipalities, localities. Then, in some localities, household targeting was used to select households based on poverty criteria.

At the beginning, all rural areas in all seventeen departments of Nicaragua were eligible for the program. The focus on rural areas reflected the distribution of poverty in the country: of the 48 percent of Nicaraguans designated as poor in 1998, 75 percent lived in rural areas (World Bank 2001). For the first phase, the government selected the departments of Madriz and Matagalpa from the central region on the basis of poverty and their capacity to implement the program. This region was the only one that showed worsening poverty between 1998 and 2001, a period during which both urban and rural poverty rates were declining nationally (World Bank 2003). In 1998 approximately 80 percent of the rural population of Madriz and Matagalpa were poor, and half of those were extremely poor (Maluccio 2005). These departments were less than a day's drive from RPS headquarters in the capital, Managua. They also had reasonably good coverage of schools and, to a lesser extent, of health posts (Arcia 1999), reducing the share of RPS resources needed to increase services (Maluccio, Murphy, and Regalía 2006).

During the next stage of geographic targeting, the RPS team chose six (of twenty) municipalities based on similar poverty criteria used at the department level. The last stage was designed to select appropriate localities from these six municipalities. A marginality index was constructed, and an index score was calculated for all fifty-nine localities. The index was a weighted average of a set of proxy poverty indicators (including family size, access to potable water, access to latrines, and illiteracy rates) in which higher index scores were associated with more impoverished areas (Arcia 1999). During the first stage of the first phase, forty-two localities with the highest scores were deemed eligible to receive the program and formed the impact evaluation area of the first phase.

The initial design called for geographic targeting in these localities—that is, all resident households were eligible to receive the transfers. Nevertheless, about 2.5 percent were excluded because they were deemed to have substantial resources by, for example, owning land or a pickup truck (Maluccio 2005). Another 6.8 percent were excluded for other reasons, such as having a single, able-bodied member or falsifying information. Finally, about 6,000 households were included as beneficiaries at the end of 2000.

To explore the effectiveness of geographic combined with household-level targeting, in mid-2001 RPS incorporated an additional 4,000 households from the remaining seventeen localities, based on a proxy means test. A model predicting households' per capita expenditures in rural areas was estimated using information from the 1998 Living Standards Measurement Survey. The RPS team designed a questionnaire to collect the information needed to register beneficiaries for the program and to apply the proxy means test. In the seventeen targeted localities, households whose predicted per capita expenditures were above a certain threshold were excluded from the program. Unintentionally, the threshold chosen for the application of the proxy means test nearly coincided with the country's official poverty line.

In the second phase, with the adoption of a consumption-based poverty map for rural areas, which was consistent with the country's official poverty map, the RPS program strengthened geographic targeting. Following a thorough analysis of the strengths and weaknesses of the proxy means test methodology, per household targeting would only be applied in localities with predicted incidence of extreme poverty of less than 45 percent.

Compliance and Payments

Households eligible for the program could receive conditional cash transfers for three years. This limitation was based on concerns about the program's fiscal sustainability; indeed, impact evaluation results suggested that some of the demand constraints households faced were not overcome in three years, especially in education.

In the first phase, households received a cash transfer (*bono alimentario*) of $224 per year, paid in six installments on a bimonthly basis. The size of the transfer did not depend on the size of the household. Receipt depended on attending the educational workshops held every other month and taking all children younger than six years old to scheduled preventive health care appointments. In the second phase, this transfer decreased to $168 in the first year, $145 in the second, and $126 in the third, last year of eligibility.

Cash transfers could be collected only by a designated household representative. In almost all cases, the RPS appointed the mother to this role, given the preponderance of evidence worldwide that resources controlled by women show higher returns for the well-being of children and the entire family. Cash payments were every second month, and mothers were required to show photo identification, bar-code program cards. All children enrolled in the program were linked to their mother's bar code. *Promotoras* and local program representatives organized and assisted the women at payment posts in each municipality. Health service providers and schoolteachers recorded households' compliance with program requirements on ad hoc RPS forms. The RPS team regularly collected these and recorded the data in a management information system, which was the basis for payment. Overall, the frequency of payments was regular.

In the first two years, approximately 10 percent of beneficiaries were penalized at least once and therefore did not receive one or both transfers (*bono escolar* and *bono alimentario*). Approximately 5 percent voluntarily left the program, either by dropping out or by leaving the program area (Maluccio and Flores 2005). Fewer than 1 percent were expelled during the first two years for reasons such as repeated failure to comply with program requirements, failure to collect the cash transfer for two consecutive periods, more than twenty-seven unexcused school absences during the school year, and false reporting.

A full listing of program requirements during the first phase, including those planned but ultimately not enforced, by type of household is presented in table 11-1. When it was learned that some, but not all, schools practiced automatic promotion, enforcement of the grade promotion condition was deemed unfair and was dropped. Similarly, when there were delays in vaccine delivery, the up-to-date vaccination condition was eliminated, as was the punishment for children who did not show adequate weight gain. These changes highlight the importance of careful program design and the need for flexibility in program implementation (Maluccio and Flores 2005).

Supply Side: Payment

To understand the degree of innovation brought about by the RPS performance-based payment program, it is important to analyze the incentive structure providers faced in 2000, before the program, and to compare the changes introduced with the trends of the sectorwide health reform.

Before the program started, preventive health care services were underused, especially by the poor. Services were provided by understaffed and chronically

Table 11-1. *Requirements in Phase One of the RPS in Nicaragua,
by Type of Household*

Program requirement	No targeted children (A)	Children ages 0–5 (B)	Children 7–13 who have not completed fourth grade (C)	(B + C)
Attend bimonthly health education workshops	✓	✓	✓	✓
Bring children to prescheduled health care appointments either monthly (younger than two years) or bimonthly (two to five years)		✓		✓
Adequate weight gain for children under five[a]		✓		✓
Enrollment in grades one to four of all targeted children in the household			✓	✓
Regular attendance (85 percent) of all targeted children in the household[b]			✓	✓
Promotion at end of school year[c]			✓	✓
Delivery of the cash transfer from the family to the teacher			✓	✓
Up-to-date vaccination for all children younger than five[b]		✓		✓

Source: Maluccio and Flores (2005).
a. Discontinued in phase two, starting in 2003.
b. No more than five absences every two months without a valid excuse.
c. Not enforced.

underfunded Ministry of Health centers. The ministry decided on budget allocations according to historical trends, with no needs-based planning or budgeting process. Public health providers were expected to cover wide geographic areas with inadequate reimbursement even for travel costs and with no incentives to extend coverage to more people. In addition, the ministry had no experience in contracting private providers. The two measures introduced by the RPS—contracting providers and aligning payments with measurable targets—were therefore dramatic changes with far-reaching effects.

In parallel, the Ministry of Health began a broader reform of the public sector in 2001, with mixed results. Targeted at improving the way medical care was organized and financed, the reform effort aimed to improve budgeting arrangements, provide incentives to improve the tracking of funds, and link financial rewards and sanctions to the use of funds. The Ministry of Health, regional health authorities, also called the Local System of Integrated Health Care (SILAIS), and health centers signed annual management agreements. These contracts specified certain actions to be taken, goals to be achieved, and budgets to be allocated at the facility level. Although the contracts were supposed to provide incentives to improve local performance, the implementation of financial rewards and sanctions so far has not been systematic. The expansion of health coverage to remote areas by contracting NGOs has also not been much of a success. What the reform has delivered, however, is better execution by SILAIS and health centers of the programmed budget, better management of commitments, and the development of monitoring mechanisms.

Two considerations follow. The RPS scheme for delivering services in underserved areas went well beyond what, at this stage, broader health sector reform has achieved. By piloting outsourced services, the program proved the feasibility of quickly overcoming capacity constraints to access health services. By paying providers based on performance, the RPS demonstrated an effective mechanism to increase access to and improve the quality of basic health services. Unfortunately, the RPS model has not yet gained enough political and institutional support to be included as part of a sectorwide strategy. This may be due, in part, to the fact that RPS was never housed within the Ministry of Health, so the health sector never fully owned the program.

To constructively engage the government in considering institutionalizing RPS as a health strategy, future research should address an important issue not discussed here: the relative cost-effectiveness of RPS-like schemes for delivering services compared to other alternatives, such as direct delivery of services by the Ministry of Health, with or without demand-side incentives.

Choice of Service Provider

The Ministry of the Family and the Ministry of Health were jointly responsible for the selection of health service providers through an international competitive bidding process. More than one provider could be contracted for a municipality with a large population. The program contracted the service of private agencies and NGOs; the providers selected were trained and certified by SILAIS.

Contract Terms

The contract specified a unit cost for each preventive health service, such as prenatal care. The amount a provider was paid was determined by multiplying the number of people served by the unit cost of the service provided. The program paid providers for the services offered, and the Ministry of Health paid for inputs like vaccines and micronutrients. Health care providers were paid every second or third month, depending on the municipality.

Providers conducted an initial analysis of the coverage of services to be offered in their assigned localities. With the help of the *promotoras,* they surveyed all households to accomplish the following:

—Validate the household-level demographic information collected through an RPS population census questionnaire,
—Identify the final universe of households to be served with a final estimation of the amount in the contract signed with the Ministry of the Family,
—Enroll households, and
—Establish a baseline for the services to be provided.

This baseline allowed the RPS team to determine the services each household member would need. It shared this information with the Ministry of Health to ensure an adequate supply of inputs, such as vaccines and micronutrients. Providers were paid a fee of about $9.30 per household for this diagnostic.

Performance and Payment

A contracted provider was paid an upfront fee of 3 percent of the entire amount of a one-year contract, with the rest paid bimonthly or quarterly as targets were met. The targets were divided into groups by beneficiary age and by categories, such as pregnant or breastfeeding women. A provider was required to offer services to between 95 and 98 percent of individuals in every group, but if it missed this target for one group, it could still be paid for services to the other groups. If targets were missed for reasons outside a provider's control, an appeal could succeed in reinstating a payment after an RPS team verified the reasons. A provider was also considered in compliance with the contract if it met with household members but was unable to deliver a service such as a vaccination because the Ministry of Health did not provide the vaccine on time. These situations became relatively rare as the program got under way. Although demand-side and supply-side incentives may not be enough to ensure a stable supply of vaccines, one reason the vaccines were more available as the program progressed might be that the incentives motivated providers to pressure suppliers of the vaccine—that is, the Ministry of Health. Providers also served households not enrolled in the RPS program but in the same localities and could be paid up to an additional 10 percent for doing so.

To verify targets, the RPS team supplied providers with ad hoc forms for each household, to be signed when a service was provided. The RPS team periodically collected these forms to assess both households' compliance with program conditions and providers' attainment of targets. Payments were then issued by the Ministry of the Family, usually within two months.

Every six months, the RPS team randomly checked a sample of providers, households, and individual beneficiaries to verify that the information that the health care providers submitted was accurate. Discovery of false reporting of information triggered a suspension of payments, and repeated false reporting terminated the contract with the health provider. Additionally, twice a year, a firm of independent external auditors performed random checks of the records of a representative sample of providers, localities, households, and individuals.

The risk of providers losing payments by not meeting targets seemed a real threat at the start of the program, but in practice, providers always complied with the 95 to 98 percent target and received full payment. Some of this success can be attributed to the program's outreach effort, such as involving *promotoras* to organize women to come for health checkups. Providers also sometimes used their own resources to mobilize schoolteachers and community leaders and to buy radio airtime to spread the program's message.

Providers subcontracted health care teams whose members were paid on average 30 to 50 percent more than the Ministry of Health personnel operating in the same municipalities. Teams operating in the most difficult terrain also received additional financial incentives. The annual cost per household for the services provided varied substantially across municipalities, with a 2005 average across all municipalities of $134.

In localities where demand-side transfers to beneficiary households stopped in 2003 but the supply of health services did not, the pay-for-performance nature of the providers' contract did not change. At first, providers continued to be paid on compliance with the 95 to 98 percent coverage target by group, but over time this changed: providers were still paid according to performance, but also according to population covered. Despite the withdrawal of demand-side transfers and changes in the terms of the contract described, preventive health service use rates remained very high eight to ten months after cash transfers were discontinued (IFPRI 2004).

Results

The original RPS design included a rigorous impact evaluation strategy in part because the two-phase IDB loan required achieving, during the first phase, a set of quantitative triggers as preconditions for the second phase. These triggers included targets that were expressed in terms of net impacts: changes in the treatment group compared to changes in a control group, known as "difference in difference." The RPS impact evaluation was therefore expected to rely on a robust design that included a control group and both a baseline and follow-up surveys to enable estimating this difference in difference. Both the government and the IDB wanted to learn as much as possible from the implementation of such of an innovative intervention, which was among the first of its type in a low-income country.

IFPRI and the government carried out the impact evaluation in close coordination, which showed strong ownership and commitment. Continuous IDB support complemented these efforts. A baseline survey in 2000 was followed by other surveys in 2001, 2002, and 2004, and a qualitative evaluation was carried out in 2003.

Overall, the RPS impact evaluation strategy was one of the most comprehensive and well executed among all social program impact evaluations carried out in Latin America and the Caribbean and one of the best of CCT programs worldwide. It also proved that an impact evaluation of its caliber could be conducted in a low-income country at a reasonable cost. Five key factors contributed to the success of the evaluation:

—A team of dedicated external consultants with sound analytical skills and the capacity to lead survey fieldwork,

—The capacity and experience of the local counterpart team that carried out survey fieldwork under the supervision of external consultants,

—The dedication of the external team to transfer knowledge to the local RPS team,

—The careful planning of all the evaluation stages from design through implementation, and

—The RPS team's commitment to stick with the planned evaluation design and implementation plans.

Such an evaluation would not have been possible had the program's execution not been consistently coherent and successful. This factor is too often taken for granted. Off-track program execution is the main determinant of an ineffective impact evaluation.

The methodological approach of the evaluation differed in the first and second phases (Maluccio and Flores 2005). The first used the randomization of localities in treatment and control groups, chosen through the transparent process of a lottery at a public event. The design of the second phase was quasi-experimental, with control localities selected in areas where the RPS did not plan to expand. This made the design less robust than randomization, but it was the only design deemed feasible. Because the evaluation of the first phase showed that the program could deliver important impacts, excluding localities by a lottery in the second phase was considered not ethically appropriate.

During its first phase, the RPS had positive double-difference estimated average effects on a broad range of indicators and outcomes. Where it did not, the result was often due to similar, though smaller, improvements in the control group. Almost all estimated effects were greater for the poorest households, often reflecting their lower starting points. As a result, the program reduced inequality across expenditure classes for a variety of outcomes (Maluccio and Flores 2005): the average net impact on total annual household expenditures per capita was 18 percent. Most of this increase was spent on food and resulted in an improvement in the diet of the beneficiaries.

In terms of health outcomes, between 2000 and 2001, the RPS induced an average net increase of 16.4 percentage points among children under three who were receiving preventive health care (Maluccio and Flores 2005). Between 2000 and 2002, the net increase was "only" 8.4 percentage points, largely as a result of continued improvement in the control group. The services provided by the RPS, as measured by process indicators such as whether a child was weighed or a health card was updated, improved to an even greater extent, especially among the extremely poor (see table 11-2). The average net impact was 13.1 percentage points, but among extremely poor households it was 18.8. Participation by children between the ages of three and five in preventive health checkups also increased substantially.

Vaccination rates climbed more than 30 percentage points to above 70 percent in the intervention areas between 2000 and 2002 (see table 11-3). A smaller increase was observed in control areas. These results are particularly striking when compared to Demographic and Health Survey figures showing coverage in rural areas declining from 68 percent in 1998 to 60 percent in 2001 (Maluccio and Flores 2005). It is likely that the Ministry of Health's supply of vaccines to providers in RPS municipalities also increased the availability of vaccines for public health units in the control localities. Given the RPS municipalities' initial vaccination coverage, it is entirely plausible to attribute at least some part of this improvement in both treatment and control localities to the RPS.

The biggest impacts on service use in both education and health were observed among very poor households (IFPRI 2003). The increased use of health services, combined with improvements in diet, led to a 5.5 percentage point decline in

Table 11-2. *Average Effect of RPS on Children from Birth to Three Years of Age in Nicaragua, by Poverty Status*[a]

Group	Extremely poor	Poor	Nonpoor
Taken to health control in the last six months			
Double difference, 2001–2000	17.5*	20.6*	6.6
	(9.0)	(8.8)	(9.4)
Double difference, 2002–2000	15.2*	6.5	−9.1
	(8.3)	(6.4)	(8.6)
Weighed in the last six months			
Double difference, 2001–2000	29.9***	23.5***	13.0
	(9.6)	(8.9)	(12.1)
Double difference, 2002–2000	18.8**	7.3	8.3
	(9.5)	(9.1)	(13.1)

Source: Maluccio and Flores (2005) using Nicaraguan RPS evaluation data.

a. Standard errors correct for heteroskedasticity and allow for clustering at the *comarca* level and are shown in parentheses (StataCorp 2001). Analysis is based on all children newborn to three years old in 706 households in the intervention group and 653 households in the control group in each year.

***$p > 0.01$
**$p > 0.05$
*$p > 0.10$

Table 11-3. *Average Effect of RPS on Percentage of Children Twelve to Twenty-Three Months of Age with Updated Vaccinations in Nicaragua*[a]

Survey round	Intervention	Control	Difference
Follow-up, 2002	71.4	69.4	2.0
	[91]	[121]	(6.0)
Follow-up, 2001	81.9	72.8	9.1
	[105]	[114]	(7.1)
Baseline, 2000	38.9	41.5	−2.6
	[139]	[123]	(9.2)
Difference, 2001–2000	43.1***	31.3***	11.7
	(7.1)	(6.8)	(9.8)
Difference, 2002–2000	32.6***	28.0***	4.6
	(7.2)	(8.5)	(11.0)

Source: Maluccio and Flores (2005) using Nicaraguan RPS evaluation data.

a. Standard errors correcting for heteroskedasticity and allowing for clustering at the *comarca* level are shown in parentheses (StataCorp 2001). Analysis is based on all children twelve to twenty-three months old in 706 households in the intervention group and 653 households in the control group in each year (number of children is shown in brackets).

***$p > 0.01$

Table 11-4. *Effect of RPS on Percentage of Children under Five Who Are Stunted in Nicaragua*[a]

Survey round	Intervention	Control	Difference
Follow-up, 2002	36.5	41.7	−5.2
	[469]	[518]	(4.7)
Baseline, 2000	39.8	39.5	0.3
	[512]	[483]	(4.9)
Difference, 2002–2000	−3.4***	2.2	−5.5*
	(1.3)	(2.8)	(3.0)

Source: Maluccio and Flores (2005) using Nicaraguan RPS evaluation data.

a. Height-for-age z score < −2.00. Standard errors correcting for heteroskedasticity and allowing for cluster-ing at the *comarca* level are shown in parentheses (StataCorp 2001). Analysis is based on all children newborn to three years old in 706 households in the intervention group and 653 households in the control group in each year.

***$p > 0.01$

*$p > 0.10$

stunting among children under five, more than one and a half times the national rate's decrease between 1998 and 2001 (see table 11-4). Very few programs in the world have rigorously demonstrated such a rapid and substantial decline in stunting (Maluccio and Flores 2005).

Between 2000 and 2002, RPS improved the distribution of iron supplements and antiparasite medicines to these same children. The dramatically high rates of anemia did not improve, however. The qualitative evaluation found that although they understood the value of supplements, mothers did not always administer them for a variety of reasons, such as children simply did not like them or they induced vomiting or diarrhea (Adato and Roopnaraine 2004). The qualitative evaluation showed that beneficiaries viewed preventive health services favorably and found the presentation of health education materials simple and accessible. Putting into practice what was presented during the health sessions proved more difficult. Beneficiaries greatly valued the quality and easy access to health ser-vices and the "good treatment" received from health care providers (Adato and Roopnaraine 2004).

The program's second phase, with average transfers reduced by 30 percent mainly for fiscal sustainability considerations, was about as effective as the first in terms of increasing the use of health services, although the measurement of results was less certain because of the change in design (IFPRI 2004). After households stopped receiving transfers but continued receiving preventive health care, ser-vice use remained around the peak reached in 2002 and even improved on some indicators, such as vaccination rates. These results can be interpreted in very different ways. It could be argued, for example, that the RPS generated, at least in the short term (eight to ten months after transfers were stopped), a lasting effect on service use. It could also be said, however, that demand subsidies might not be needed and that setting up an effective delivery scheme might be enough. For the same households, use of education services declined after transfers were discontinued, halving the net gains in school enrollment during the program's first phase. One possible interpretation suggests that the cost of sending children to school is higher than the cost associated with health checkups.

In the second phase, the program generated a net average impact of 5 percentage points in the use of family planning methods among females between twelve and forty-nine years old. The impact was three times greater among women between thirty and forty. The qualitative evaluation stresses the variation across localities, mainly related to religion, with less support for family planning in evangelical localities (Adato and Roopnaraine 2004).

Program impacts on the use of maternal care services were rather modest, mainly because of improvements in the control group. In the first phase, the impact on pregnant women having at least one prenatal checkup was estimated at 24.5 percentage points. This declined to 15.1 percentage points in the second phase. A marginally significant net impact of 4.6 percentage points was seen among women who had at least one postnatal checkup (from an extremely low initial coverage of 8.3 percent) in the second phase.

Role of Government

The Nicaraguan Emergency Social Investment Fund designed and successfully executed the program's first phase. ESIF's institutional structure, accounting systems, and nationwide presence at the local level provided an excellent platform for development of the RPS program. The program's intended activities bore little similarity to ESIF's core activities, however, making the upfront investment of time and resources for the RPS team very high. Transfers and supply-side interventions did not start until the end of the first year of operation. The first-year cost-transfer ratio—the administration and private costs associated with a one-unit transfer to beneficiaries—was 2.54. That is, $2.54 was spent to transfer $1 of benefits to eligible households either as demand subsidies or as health care services. The cost-transfer ratio improved dramatically throughout the course of the program (Caldés and Maluccio 2005), reaching a low of about $0.20 by 2005.

Before the second phase, the RPS team was moved from ESIF to the Ministry of the Family to institutionalize the program within a line ministry and strengthen coordination among the Ministry of Health, the Ministry of the Family, and the Ministry of Education. This coordination remained patchy, and the program suffered a setback in autonomy and in its plans to reduce administrative costs.

At the start, the Ministry of Health considered RPS as a headache and agreed only reluctantly to IDB's suggestion of outsourcing health services to reach remote localities. Relations between RPS and the ministry remained tense during the first phase for several reasons, including the ministry's increased workload and the higher wages of contracted providers. At the central level, differences arose over the ceiling of $90 per household per year imposed by the Ministry of Health, despite wanting the RPS to provide more services. The final cost was about 50 percent higher.

By the second phase, relations between the Ministry of Health and the Ministry of the Family improved: information, training, and part of the resources were shared, and each side appreciated the expanded coverage in remote areas. Despite this progress and the impact evaluation results, however, the model of private services provision is far from being institutionalized in the Nicaraguan health sector. It is regrettable that current Ministry of Health budgets earmark no resources to contract providers for RPS localities beyond the program's five years. For extremely poor households in RPS areas, therefore, access to maternal and child care services will once again become elusive. Had the Ministry of Health been given more ownership over the program from the beginning, the increased support within the health sector might well have led to improved institutionalization and continuity.

Conclusions

The difficulty in disentangling the individual impacts of demand-side and supply-side incentives aside, the RPS evaluation clearly shows that combining the two can significantly increase the use of health services among poor households and improve health outcomes. An evaluation about ten months after demand-side incentives had been stopped in certain areas revealed that use rates for preventive health care services remained high. This might be because the program strategy dramatically improved provider outreach activities and thus the access of poor households to health services, reducing the costs of time and travel to reach delivery points. It is possible, therefore, that a well-targeted strategy of supply-side, performance incentives could, on its own, be enough to achieve and maintain high levels of health care service use among poor rural populations in Nicaragua. The RPS evaluation shows that this conclusion holds among poor households that have benefited from a relatively long period (three years) of education on the importance of preventive health care, alongside demand-side financial incentives, at least ten months after the incentives had been discontinued. The results, though, cannot exclude that, even after their removal, demand-side incentives continue to exert, at least in the short term, a positive impact on service use. In considering RPS-like approaches, future research efforts should be devoted to unbundling the bundle of incentives and assessing the relative contribution of supply versus demand incentives.

References

Adato, Michelle, and Terry Roopnaraine. 2004. "Sistema de evaluación de la Red de Protección Social de Nicaragua: Un análisis social de la 'Red de Protección Social' (RPS) en Nicaragua." Washington: International Food Policy Research Institute.

Arcia, G. 1999. "Proyecto de Red de Protección Social: Focalización de la fase piloto." Report submitted to the Inter-American Development Bank. Washington.

Caldés, Natalia, and John A. Maluccio. 2005. "The Cost of Conditional Cash Transfers." *Journal of International Development* 17 (2): 151–68.

Eichler, Rena. 2006. "Can 'Pay for Performance' Increase Utilization by the Poor and Improve the Quality of Health Services?" Discussion paper for the first meeting of the Working Group on Performance-Based Incentives. Center for Global Development, Washington, February 7.

IFPRI (International Food Policy Research Institute). 2001. "Evaluation System for the Pilot Phase of Nicaraguan Red de Protección Social: Baseline 2000." Report submitted to the Red de Protección Social. Washington.

———. 2003. "Sistema de evaluación de la fase piloto de la Red de Protección Social de Nicaragua: Evaluación de impacto 2000–2002." Report submitted to the Red de Protección Social. Washington.

———. 2004. "Informe final sistema de evaluación de la Red de Protección Social (RPS): MIFAMILIA, Nicaragua: Evaluación del impacto: 2000–04." Report submitted to the Red de Protección Social. Washington.

Maluccio, John. 2005. "Coping with the Coffee Crisis in Central America: The Role of the Nicaraguan Red de Protección Social." Food Consumption and Nutrition Division Discussion Paper 188. Washington: International Food Policy Research Institute.

Maluccio, John, and Raphael Flores. 2005. "Impact Evaluation of the Pilot Phase of the Nicaraguan Red de Protección Social." Research Report 141. Washington: International Food Policy Research Institute.

Maluccio, John, Alexis Murphy, and Fernandino Regalía. 2006. "Does Supply Matter? Initial Supply Conditions and the Effectiveness of Conditional Cash Transfers for Schooling in Nicaragua." Washington: Inter-American Development Bank.

Schady, Norbert, and María Caridad Araujo. 2006. "Cash Transfers, Conditions, School Enrollment, and Child Work: Evidence from a Randomized Experiment in Ecuador." Unpublished manuscript. Washington: World Bank, Development Economics Research Group.

StataCorp. 2001. Stata Statistical Software: Release 6. College Station, Texas: StataCorp LP.

World Bank. 2001. *Nicaragua Poverty Assessment: Challenges and Opportunities for Poverty Reduction*. Report 20488-NI. Washington.

———. 2003. *Nicaragua Poverty Assessment: Raising Welfare and Reducing Vulnerability*. Report 26128-NI. Washington.

12

Worldwide: Incentives for Tuberculosis Diagnosis and Treatment

Alexandra Beith, Rena Eichler, and Diana Weil

Highlights

Many tuberculosis programs incorporate material (food) and financial performance-based incentives for patients, providers, or both.

Findings from a combination of rigorous evaluations and data from routine program monitoring suggest that performance incentives can improve both case detection and treatment adherence.

Performance incentives applied to tuberculosis contain lessons for treatment of other extended-duration and chronic conditions.

The authors express their sincere appreciation to Sangeeta Mookherji for devoting her time and energy to providing detailed comments and references and for sharing her knowledge with us. We would like to thank Irina Danilova, Wieslaw Jacubowiak, Knut Lönnroth, Tom Mohr, Mukund Uplekar, Tatyana Vinichenko, Otabek Rajabov, and I. D. Rusen for providing details through discussion and by responding to drafts of this paper. Gratitude is also expressed to the U.S. Agency for International Development, Management Sciences for Health, World Health Organization, and Stop TB Partnership for support that initiated the work on the application of incentives in tuberculosis control programs between 2001 and 2003, on which this chapter draws heavily. They appreciated the support provided by Jessica Gottlieb and Aaron Pied.

Many tuberculosis (TB) control programs incorporate performance-based financial or material incentives, or both, for patients and providers with the intent of increasing the number of TB cases detected and ultimately cured. Patient incentives are frequently tied to actions that are closely linked to completing treatment. Provider incentives are tied to actions, outcome measures, or both. Findings from a few well-designed evaluations and routine reporting data from tuberculosis programs suggest that financial and material incentives can have a positive influence on the detection of tuberculosis cases and full adherence to TB treatment.

Tuberculosis remains a lethal threat to public health. The World Health Organization (WHO) estimated that nearly 9 million people developed active TB and some 1.6 million died from it in 2005. Ninety-eight percent of TB deaths occur in the developing world, and the majority of those affected are the poor and vulnerable, including those with compromised immune systems such as from HIV/AIDS and malnutrition (WHO 2007). Recently, TB has been declared an emergency in Africa, and it is a grave concern in parts of Eastern Europe and Central Asia for a number of reasons, including rising incidence, HIV-associated tuberculosis, and increasing prevalence of multidrug-resistant tuberculosis. In contrast, in most of Asia, the Middle East, the Americas, and Western Europe, economic development and stronger responses to TB have contributed to a decline in both prevalence and mortality.

To reach the Millennium Development Goal of reversing the incidence of tuberculosis and the Stop TB Partnership targets for 2015 of reducing mortality and prevalence rates by 50 percent, it will be necessary to nearly double the detection of TB cases in Africa, increase treatment success rates to at least 85 percent, and expand implementation of strategies to address HIV-associated and multidrug-resistant tuberculosis. A new Stop TB Strategy and the Global Plan to Stop TB 2006–2015 are providing the frameworks for scaling up these efforts. Evidence suggests that performance incentives can contribute to these goals.

Here we provide an overview of performance-based financial and material incentives that are being used in a range of countries to improve the detection of tuberculosis and the completion of treatment. We draw on the collaborative work of the Stop TB Partnership, the World Health Organization, the World Bank, the Rational Pharmaceutical Management Plus (RPM Plus) project managed by Management Sciences for Health, with financing by the U.S. Agency for International Development (USAID) and other sources.[1] Evidence is drawn substantially

1. For an overview, see www.msh.org/projects/rpmplus/3.5.5.htm [October 2008].

from information collected through four surveys of TB incentive interventions conducted by the collaborative in 2001 and 2003 and the RPM Plus program in 2004 and 2005.[2]

Evidence suggests that incentives can be valuable in implementing the components of the Stop TB Strategy. Although it is difficult, given the available evidence, to attribute changes in performance fully to the incentives, experience indicates that performance incentives for patients and providers can help to support increased detection of cases and contribute directly to an improvement in treatment completion rates. Reviewing cases of performance incentives in TB programs reveals the importance of careful design and implementation, particularly involving the distribution of money or food.

For this discussion, *incentive* is defined as "all financial or material rewards that patients and/or providers receive, conditional on their explicitly measured performance or behavior."[3]

Context of TB Control

Tuberculosis is predominately a disease of the poor, making adherence to the extended course of treatment a considerable challenge. Without effective strategies to ensure adherence to treatment and appropriate patient management, the danger of developing drug-resistant forms of tuberculosis increases. The newly enhanced Stop TB Strategy builds on knowledge of what is needed to deliver effective tuberculosis care in the increasingly complex environment of drug-resistant TB and HIV/AIDS co-infection.

Tuberculosis thrives in the context of poverty. In addition to its impact on an individual's ability to work and earn a living, the costs of seeking accurate diagnosis and treatment can be considerable for low-income households. TB patients face substantial costs before diagnosis in that they often consult several public and private providers before and in the process of being diagnosed (Hanson, Weil, and Floyd 2006). Although most public services provide tests and TB drugs free of

2. This used the broader terminology *incentives and enablers* to categorize and analyze motivators for patients and providers to overcome obstacles to detecting TB and adhering to treatment. *Incentive* was defined as "incites someone to determination or action, introduces additional motivations to achieve existing performance objectives or to achieve higher performance standards." *Enabler* was defined as "makes something possible, practical, or easy; allows action based on existing motivations or to achieve performance standards or goals within existing systems frameworks." *Motivators* could be financial, material, nonfinancial, and nonmaterial.

3. This definition is similar to that of Robert Town and his colleagues (2004). It has been adapted slightly to fit the TB control context.

charge, other direct and opportunity costs pose barriers to accessing TB services and treatment, especially for poor rural and marginalized urban patients (such as slum dwellers, migrants, the homeless). In many cases, patients resort to borrowing money or selling assets (Nhlema and others 2004, cited in Stop TB/WHO 2006). Many of the performance-based financial and material incentive schemes targeted at patients are designed to help compensate for these costs, thus overcoming a considerable obstacle faced by poor patients.

Adherence to at least six months of treatment is a challenge. Tuberculosis can be cured with a cocktail of three or four drugs that cost as little as $14 to $18 per patient. However, adherence often poses a challenge because treatment for patients with drug-sensitive disease is six to eight months and involves repeated interactions with health services. Challenges are on both the patient (demand) and provider (supply) sides. Without proper health education on the risks of stopping treatment early and other motivators to encourage continued treatment, patients may stop taking drugs when they start to feel better. Unreliable drug supply, poor prescribing practices, and inadequate patient management can also result in inappropriate TB treatment.

Drug resistance is an increasing concern. In addition to failing to cure the patient, poor adherence contributes to development of strains of the bacterium that are resistant to treatment. Strains that are resistant to at least the two core anti-TB drugs, called multidrug-resistant tuberculosis, are an increasing threat to global efforts to control tuberculosis. Although it is a more severe problem in some countries, multidrug-resistant TB has been documented in nearly every country in the world, with nearly half a million cases each year (Stop TB/WHO 2006). Drug-resistant TB is usually treatable but requires two years of treatment that is far more expensive and potentially toxic to patients.[4]

Core Elements

The core elements of an effective TB control program are well established. In 2000 the WHO World Health Assembly agreed on 2005 targets for both detection of cases (70 percent of new smear-positive cases) and completion of treatment (successful treatment of 85 percent of those detected) with the goal of decreasing the global TB burden. Where HIV is absent, reaching these targets should lead to a substantial decrease in prevalence rates and an annual decrease in incidence of about 5 to 10 percent (Stop TB/WHO 2006).

4. See WHO fact sheets, www.who.int/mediacentre/factsheets/fs104/en/#hiv [October 2008].

DOTS—directly observed treatment/therapy short course, the internationally recommended approach to controlling TB—underpins efforts to improve tuberculosis control worldwide and reach these targets. Since 1995, DOTS has been scaled up globally, with more than 20 million patients treated under this approach by the end of 2004. It incorporates five elements: political commitment, case detection through quality-assured bacteriology, short-course chemotherapy and patient support, a regular supply of quality-assured drugs, and routine systems of reporting, monitoring, and impact evaluation. At the end of 2003, more than three-quarters of the global population lived in countries that had adopted DOTS (Stop TB/WHO 2006).

In 2006, building on the successes of DOTS, the World Health Organization launched an expanded strategy called the Stop TB Strategy, which incorporates additional policy and implementation innovations to address TB/HIV, multidrug resistance, and the challenges of reaching new populations and providers, empowering communities, and promoting research. The Stop TB Strategy and Global Plan 2006–2015, which aims to reduce the suffering associated with TB and increase equitable access to care, dovetails with the objectives of universal access for HIV prevention, treatment, and care.

In this context, performance incentives can have an impact on both the supply side and the demand side of TB care, treatment, and prevention. Incentives can be applied to improve public health outcomes by helping to cure infectious patients and increase access and by reducing the suffering of affected individuals by encouraging and enabling patients to seek care early and get effective care.

Directly observed treatment is a core element of TB control programs. The DOT standard requires that a health worker, community volunteer, or family member supports and observes patients taking their anti-TB medicines. This need emerged from experience in South Asia, the United States, and elsewhere, where high default rates and the risk of drug-resistant disease attributable to intermittent or incomplete treatment led to concern that more direct support was needed. Effective DOT can ensure patient adherence and cure and does reduce the risk of multidrug resistance, but it entails a high level of patient-provider contacts, which can impose substantial costs on the patient.

Treatment Options

There is a range of approaches to treating and managing tuberculosis. In some countries, patients are hospitalized during the first two months of treatment and attend health services on an ambulatory basis for the remaining six months. In most of the world, however, TB patients receive treatment on an ambulatory basis. During that phase, patients can attend a clinic or, as many increasingly are, participate in a community-based program in which community workers, volunteers, or family members provide the necessary support to ensure that the patient adheres to the treatment schedule. Because the success of this approach and the DOT model rely on the patient and provider sustaining certain behaviors over the course of the treatment, performance incentives are a promising strategy.

Existing incentives, however, can discourage the actions necessary for full TB treatment. One of the many reasons that TB programs do not always achieve performance targets is that the many people who form a tuberculosis control system may not contribute effectively to case detection, treatment completion, and cure. That is, providers may not always follow guidelines for appropriate detection and treatment, even when they have the knowledge, tools, and environment to do so. Confounding the problem is that patients may not always seek care or stay on the recommended treatment regimen, even when drugs are available and the importance of completing treatment has been communicated and is clear.

Patient barriers to accessing, initiating, and completing TB treatment are a greater challenge for the poor, for whom performance-based financial or material incentives such as food, transportation subsidies, and money may be effective at reducing the direct and opportunity costs of treatment. By reducing obstacles, performance incentives encourage individuals to seek care and follow treatment.

Various factors may motivate (or demotivate) providers. Providing TB services is demanding because the extended course of treatment requires substantial efforts from health workers to ensure that patients adhere to the treatment schedule. Several factors discourage providers from providing effective diagnosis and care of tuberculosis patients.

—The salaries of public sector health workers often do not depend on the quality of their work, the quantity of services provided, or the results achieved. The resources needed to reach out to community members or to follow up on defaulters are often not available.

—In settings where public sector providers also run private clinics, tuberculosis patients may be unappealing to treat because they are less likely to pay fees when drugs are available in public facilities at no charge.

—Private for-profit providers in developing countries often receive fees for each service they provide. This may drive them to keep a fee-paying patient with tuberculosis rather than refer the patient to other providers to be accurately diagnosed and treated.

—At the level of health institutions (clinics and hospitals), funding is often based on a budget that covers the costs of inputs rather than being linked to health results achieved. Such an incentive justifies expenditures rather than demonstrates results.

Improving Incentives

A range of performance incentives, both financial and material, has been used successfully to improve TB results. They focus on the design of incentives, implementation, evaluation, and evidence of impact.

Patients

Patient incentives include direct payment, deposit return, food (hot meals, dry rations, or food vouchers), transportation subsidies (reimbursement, tokens, passes, or vouchers), vouchers for material goods other than food, and packages of personal hygiene products, such as shampoo. Tuberculosis patients in the United States, where the majority are low income, socially disadvantaged, and sometimes homeless, have long received financial and material incentives. In developing countries, some projects specifically target the poor (Tajikistan) or marginalized populations (Orel and Vladimir oblasts in Russia), whereas others cover all TB patients within a given region or country (Cambodia).

Patient incentives are based on performance when they depend on some required, measurable action, most commonly steps in the treatment process rather than treatment outcomes. Examples include providing food or money to patients who regularly attend a clinic to receive treatment under DOT and who complete treatment. A few patient incentive schemes require patients to assume some financial risk.

To take one example, the Bangladesh Rural Advancement Committee implemented a patient incentive scheme from 1984 to 2003 in which patients made a deposit when beginning treatment. A portion of the deposit was returned when treatment was completed. The balance was retained by the volunteer health worker who provided DOT support to the patient during treatment. The incentive program was changed in 2004, however. The patient now receives the entire deposit when the treatment is completed, and the program pays the worker.

In another case, the Perkumpulan Pemeberantasan Tuberkulosis Indonesia-Jakarta program provides patients with free drugs once they begin treatment.

A patient must sign a contract agreeing to pay the full cost of drugs taken if she or he defaults, thus providing a strong incentive to complete the treatment (Beith and others 2001).

Performance-based incentives can be designed to influence provider behavior at the levels of both the individual worker and the institution. At the individual level, incentives are aimed at improving the quality of diagnosis, expanding access to treatment by promoting outreach, reducing default rates, and encouraging completion of treatment. Incentives aimed at the team or institution level are oriented toward improving teamwork and stimulating systemic changes to improve outcomes. Payment usually is based on clearly defined measures of process or outcome, such as number of cases detected, referrals of suspected cases, patients completing treatment, or patients cured.

In the public sector, goals are to promote the extension of DOTS services beyond public facilities to ensure greater access and increased adherence. Examples of incentives targeting individual public health workers include direct payment, food packages, vouchers, and other material goods (such as briefcases, watches, soap, and so on).

Private providers have not until recent years been incorporated into a country's tuberculosis control program and have had few incentives to follow national tuberculosis guidelines. As a result, there has been considerable concern about tuberculosis drugs not being prescribed appropriately by private providers (Uplekar and others 1996; Lönnroth, Uplekar, and Blanc 2006) and about the tendency of private providers not to monitor treatment or maintain records (Lönnroth 2000; Uplekar, Pathania, and Raviglione 2001).

There is growing recognition, however, that the first contact a tuberculosis suspect has with the health care system is often with a private (whether for-profit or nonprofit) provider. This has motivated the development of public-private mix models of care including nonmonetary incentives to encourage private providers to refer suspects, or diagnosed cases, to the public health system or to supervise treatment (Ambe and others 2005; Lönnroth and others 2004; see box 12-1).

Performance-based financial and material incentives are also used to motivate provider teams or, at the organization level, to increase the number of cases detected and people cured. The theory is that incentives at the team or organization level inspire discovery and innovations at the system level, which strengthen organizations and improve effectiveness. Effectiveness depends on quality of design, management, and monitoring. Experience from existing performance-based incentive initiatives suggests some lessons about the importance of appropriate design, implementation, and evaluation of the scheme (see box 12-2).

Box 12-1. *Soft Contracts with Private Practitioners to Improve Tuberculosis Outcomes*

World Health Organization researchers reviewed fifteen public-private mix models in TB control involving national tuberculosis programs in partnership with private care providers or with not-for-profit umbrella organizations that worked with individual providers. They examined the nature of contractual relationships, quality of care, and results. In nearly all models, private providers received no formal financial payments, although they did enter contracts that enabled them to receive public sector TB drugs for free distribution to patients as well as continuing education, associated their work with a reputed national program, and ensured that they followed national guidelines and reported results to the national tuberculosis program. There were no competitive tenders. Treatment success rates were above 80 percent in thirteen initiatives and on a par with or better than national averages. TB case detection rose 10 to 36 percent. The review yielded three key conclusions:

—High treatment success rates are possible for patients receiving treatment from private providers following international standards of TB care, linked within a national DOTS-based TB program, and providing TB drugs free of charge to patients.

—Engaging private providers can increase TB case detection rates, another measure of performance in TB control.

—Informal, well-defined drugs-for-performance contracts (without direct financial payments) are a possibility when involving individual private practitioners in TB program implementation. They act as incentives for participation and are associated with good performance and improved patient and public health outcomes.

Source: Lönnroth, Uplekar, and Blanc (2006).

Stakeholder involvement is critical in the design process. Evidence suggests that consulting with patients to better understand the obstacles they face in being diagnosed and completing treatment, and with providers to better understand what is impeding them from performing optimally, may contribute to better design and increased buy-in among stakeholders. For example, in St. Petersburg, Russia, a needs assessment approach was essential to designing the incentive. Prisoners with tuberculosis who were soon to be released were asked what would motivate them most to adhere to treatment once they were back in the community. The most highly valued incentive for prisoners was assistance with obtaining a national identity card. Lack of such a card in Russia means that an individual loses opportunities for work, housing, and access to public services and has a greater likelihood of police harassment and reincarceration.[5]

5. Personal communication, Kaveh Khoshnood, Yale University, October 2004.

Box 12-2. *Incentives for Health Workers and Institutions*

The following countries offer incentives aimed at individual health workers:

—In Romania, public health workers receive gift tickets conditional on measures such as the number of new cases confirmed by microscopy and the rate of DOT in sputum-positive patients (Mookherji and Beith 2005).
    —In Honduras, public health workers receive material incentives (soap, hats, bags, towels, and so on) when program objectives are reached, such as patients regularly attending clinic-based treatment (Honduran National Tuberculosis Program response to 2004 RPM Plus survey; Mookherji and Beith 2005).

The following programs offer incentives aimed at private health care providers:

—In China, village doctors (community health workers) receive a fee for each new sputum-positive smear case that is enrolled in treatment, another when a smear exam is performed following two months of treatment, and a third when patients complete treatment (Beith and others 2001; Mookherji and others 2005; Mookherji and Beith 2005).
    —In India and the Philippines, national tuberculosis control programs supply private providers with anti-TB drugs at no cost on the condition that patients pay nothing for the drugs. Dispensing free drugs is an incentive for providers because they can charge consultation fees. In addition, providers who are known to cure TB patients develop a strong reputation as healers, which can result in higher client demand for all services.

The following programs offer incentives aimed at teams and institutions:

—In Bolivia in 2004, the goal of a national program was to inspire team-based solutions to improving program results. Payment depended on reaching service targets in rural areas, defined as the number of cured patients, home visits conducted (three per patient), community education sessions attended, and effective supervision of health promotion workers (Bolivian National Tuberculosis Program response to 2004 RPM Plus survey; Beith and others 2004; Mookherji and Beith 2005).
    —In Brazil in 2000, municipalities were paid for each patient cured and for providing access to DOT. One level of payment was for patients who self-administered the TB medicines and the other, higher amount was for those who were supervised (Beith and others 2001).
    —In the Czech Republic, nongovernmental organizations receive a monetary incentive once diagnostic tests are performed on TB suspects (L. Trnka, National Tuberculosis Program, Czech Republic response to 2005 RPM Plus survey; Mookherji and Beith 2005).
    —The Fund for Innovative DOT Expansion through Local Initiatives to Stop TB project aims to stimulate innovative approaches to increase case detection by awarding projects with second-year financing conditional on achieving scores demonstrating that patients who had had limited access were reached (personal communication, I. D. Rusen, Rena Eichler, and Alexandra Beith, June 2006).

The devil is in the details of implementation. The details of operationalizing an incentive scheme are important for programs to be able to expand to scale, ensure impact, and be sustainable. Once a performance incentive is chosen, it is critical to plan all the levels of implementation:

—Communicate the performance-based incentive scheme to recipients. Effectively communicating the new program to the people whose actions are intended to be affected is critical to success. If they do not understand it, they are unlikely to respond. For example, in El Salvador, providers did not fully understand the purpose of the patient food support, viewing it more for its nutritional benefit than for its ability to influence behavior. As a result, instead of tying it to patient adherence to treatment, they provided food to all patients, regardless of adherence (Mookherji and others 2005; Mookherji and Beith 2005).

—Decide how performance will be monitored, how performance will be reported, measured, and monitored, and who is responsible for each role. This may involve assistance to build capacity if, for example, a government department will be taking on a new function.

—Plan how the incentive will be managed. Once performance is verified, the process to move the money or material goods is critical. Schemes break down when the performance incentive is not available as promised or when recipients begin to doubt the credibility of the provider of the incentive. The Cambodia example highlights the complexity of managing food programs (see box 12-3).

—Monitor and evaluate regularly. Continuing to evaluate a scheme's effectiveness is important, as the impact of incentive schemes may wane, resulting in a need for revision. It is also critical to continue to monitor whether any unintended effects of the scheme have surfaced.

Unintended effects can be minimized with careful design and regular monitoring. One danger of offering money or food as an incentive to encourage patients to be tested or to continue treatment is that the extreme poor may react by engaging in practices that allow them to continue to qualify. Considering these potential unintended effects and establishing an ongoing monitoring system to identify and correct them are an important part of design and implementation.

In India, monitoring revealed that some patients attempted to prolong the treatment period by avoiding medicines so that they could continue to receive a monthly payment. As a result, the scheme was revised restricting payment to include a maximum six-month period from the date treatment began (Urban Poverty Alleviation Department, Cochin, India, in response to 2001 Stop TB, WHO, World Bank, and RPM Plus survey).

Box 12-3. *Cambodia: Managing Food Distribution*

Food has been provided to TB patients in Cambodia since 1994. Food packages from the World Food Program of canned fish, vegetable oil, and rice generally arrive on a monthly basis for eight months. In 2002 nearly 18,000 individuals benefited from this program. Until the end of 2002, most TB patients were hospitalized for the first two months (the intensive treatment). They received food packages weekly from the World Food Program if they remained in the hospital and continued to follow treatment. The program offset the family's costs of having to provide meals in the hospital. Outpatient patients received food support conditional on making required visits and adhering to treatment under DOT.

Cambodia has since moved to a fully ambulatory system. Food packages are conditional on continued attendance at the clinic for treatment. Some programs distribute food every month, some every two weeks.

Food Distribution

The World Food Program handles procurement and first-level distribution, and the Ministry of Health handles distribution to patients. A local firm, Khmer Express Transport, moves the food from Phnom Penh to two provincial warehouses. World Food Program staff deliver the food to outpatient departments, referral hospitals, and former district hospitals (now health centers). Health centers along the delivery routes are sometimes serviced directly. The delivery point for food is not always the same as that for medicine, and thus accessing food support implies that the patients incur additional costs. When it does not have a provincial warehouse, the World Food Program delivers the food directly from the national warehouse to the outpatient departments and referral hospitals. TB staff at health centers and former district hospitals are responsible for collecting food from health service delivery sites. The delivery point for food is the same as for TB medicines.

Monitoring

Decentralization and an increased number of food service delivery points are challenges that merit careful attention. Regular coordination between the Ministry of Health, National Tuberculosis Program, and the World Food Program has been critical. The World Food Program conducts monthly monitoring visits to check food distribution and stock levels, verify new patient lists, and review stock balance sheets. Field monitors make random spot checks during food distribution, at which time they check food ration cards against the TB register to ensure that false patients do not receive food supplements. Reporting systems related to food support (that is, keeping track of beneficiaries and leakage) follow World Food Program requirements. National coordination meetings are held on a regular basis to address operational and management concerns and to identify collaborative solutions.

Mobilizing local resources to fund timely and efficient distribution of food to peripheral health centers has become more difficult in recent years. In one province (Kampong Speu), a system has been established that uses Ministry of Health facilities and DOTS delivery points by allocating part of the budget for operating costs obtained through user fees. Health facility directors in other provinces have shown interest in this approach.

Sources: Mookherji (2005); Mookherji and Weil (2005); Mookherji and others (2003).

In Haiti, where a patient food package scheme was implemented, there was evidence of patients in control areas (without food) pressuring providers to transfer them to food support areas. This resulted in some failures since some patients were referred to pilot centers located far from their residence (Midy, Exume, and Celestin 2004; Mookherji and Beith 2005; E. Nicolas, National Tuberculosis Program, Haiti, in response to 2005 RPM Plus survey). In addition, providers involved in the patient food support scheme began to demand food, so providing food to health care workers was ultimately included in the scheme to avoid pilferage (Midy, Exume, and Celestin 2004).

In Cambodia, there were problems with "ghost" patients (treatment cards being used to obtain food packages for patients who did not have tuberculosis or were dead). The problem was overcome through effective communication and coordination among partners, more training and supervision, and tighter monitoring (Mookherji and Weil 2005).

Impact on Outcomes

The majority of tuberculosis programs known to be using performance-based financial or material incentives assess the impact of these incentives as part of regular program monitoring. Because tuberculosis programs use a standard recording and monitoring system built on routine service-based data that has been institutionalized worldwide, they have access to better information with which to monitor results than most other public health programs. Nearly all countries in the world have the estimated number of potential new tuberculosis cases and the actual number of new cases detected. Of patients who initiate treatment, those who complete it and are cured are tracked, as are those who default. This implies that TB programs can track progress in case detection and treatment completion using institutionalized information from routine monitoring.

Evaluating impact with the use of routine monitoring systems has a number of weaknesses, however. One is that multiple program-strengthening interventions may be implemented simultaneously, making it hard to attribute changes in performance fully to the incentives. Evaluations that include a control group that receives all strengthening interventions except for the incentive may be a way to overcome such weaknesses, although even these evaluations can face challenges.[6]

6. In Haiti, where a patient food package scheme was implemented in some areas, there was evidence of patients pressuring providers to transfer them from control areas, where no food was provided, to intervention areas, where food was provided (Midy, Exume, and Celestin 2004; see also Mookherji and others 2005; Mookherji and Beith 2005).

Because there are many variations on the design and implementation of incentive schemes for both providers and patients, understanding more of the details of each program and aspects of each design that contribute to success or failure is extremely useful. Few programs complement quantitative with qualitative analysis.

Evidence from Studies

A few more rigorous evaluations have been conducted in which routine monitoring data were used as well as retrospective analysis to assess the impact of performance-based incentives on TB program outcomes. These evaluations attempted to design studies that would distinctly identify the impact of incentives on performance. However, attribution is difficult because of design and implementation challenges as well as the problem of attributing changes in performance to the incentives, which is common to retrospective analyses of routine reporting data. On the patient side, findings from three evaluation studies suggest positive impacts from the incentives.

In three Russian oblasts (Ivanovo, Orel, and Vladimir), a package of interventions (food and, in some cases, travel support, clothing, or hygienic kits) was given if the patient did not interrupt treatment (see box 12-4). Default rates dropped from 15–20 percent to 2–6 percent.

In Tajikistan, vulnerable patients were given food, conditional on their adherence to treatment (see box 12-5). A treatment success rate of 89.5 percent was achieved (versus 59.4 percent for the comparison group).

In Kazakhstan, a study compared the impact of three interventions on patient adherence: patient monetary payment, hot meals for patients, and nurse outreach.[7] No single intervention was significantly more effective than another, but the combination of interventions improved treatment success by 4.7 percent.

On the provider side, findings from the few known evaluation studies also suggest a positive impact of performance incentives on referrals of suspected cases, detection of cases, and completion of treatment. Again, however, it was not possible to identify the distinct contribution of the financial and material incentives to improved performance because the studies evaluated the impact of a package of interventions.

In Bangladesh, a cost-effectiveness study of the Bangladesh Rural Advancement Committee scheme showed that TB case management using community health workers, of which the patient deposit-provider incentive payment was one

---

7. The latter, however, does not fit the definition of *incentive* used here.

Box 12-4. *Evaluations from Russia*

Since 2000, TB outpatients in the Russian oblasts of Orel and Vladimir have been provided a combination of food packages, hot meals, transport reimbursement, hygiene packages, and clothing based on their continued clinic attendance and observed treatment. When patients interrupt treatment for seven days or more, they are denied the incentive package for a week or a month depending on the territory. In 2005 the management and financing of the incentive programs were transferred to the local oblast administration.

In Vladimir (population 3,200),

—All TB outpatients receive food packages following DOT of prescribed TB drugs,
—All new TB patients are compensated for travel expenses to places of treatment depending on their clinic attendance, and
—All new TB patients receive bonus incentives (clothing, hygienic kits, and so on) when they complete an uninterrupted treatment schedule.

In Orel (population 1,200),

—TB patients in urban areas receive a hot meal or food parcels following DOT of prescribed TB drugs,
—TB patients in rural areas receive food parcels once every two weeks following two weeks of uninterrupted treatment,
—Especially vulnerable patients (70 percent of all TB patients, including the unemployed, former prisoners, migrants, homeless, those with two or more minor children, and students) receive additional food parcels every two weeks after two weeks of uninterrupted treatment,
—All patients receive hygienic kits conditional on clinic attendance and adherence to treatment, and
—Some ambulatory patients receive reimbursement for transport expenses based on clinic attendance and adherence to treatment.

Default rates in Orel and Vladimir were between 2 and 6 percent in 2004, down from between 15 and 20 percent when the program began in 1999.

The full package of social support decreased default outcomes, but the contribution of financial and material incentives cannot be distinguished from other interventions. (A recent retrospective study that included new pulmonary smear-positive and smear-negative TB patients from six Russian regions, including Orel and Vladimir, used multivariate analysis to identify the contribution of the social support package of interventions to decreasing default rates. The analysis also included other predictors of default, such as employment status, alcohol abuse, and homelessness.)

Expanding this approach nationwide may not bring similar results given that the present model is implemented in small regions with strong TB management teams that do not exist in much of the rest of the country. In addition, most regional administrations have no budgets for food and transportation subsidies for TB patients, and there are procedural and regulatory obstacles.

Box 12-5. *Evaluations from Tajikistan*

The program focuses on vulnerable patients and their families. From its initiation in 2002 until the end of 2004, the program used standard World Food Program criteria to determine who qualified as vulnerable. Criteria included the amount of arable land and number of animals owned by the family as well as the family's monthly income. Project HOPE conducted random home visits to confirm patient reports on the number of family members and the household conditions of the patient. In practice, very few TB patients were disqualified as being "not vulnerable." Moreover, the program felt that many patients who were classified as "not vulnerable" based on World Food Program criteria were vulnerable, and since 2004 the program was expanded to cover almost all TB/DOTS patients.

A population of 3,838 is served as follows:

—Food packages are provided to vulnerable patients and their families on a bimonthly basis conditional on adherence to treatments.

—Providers maintain and review treatment cards to determine adherence. Food packages contain wheat flour, vegetable oil, pulses, and salt.

—The package value is approximately $172, which, for the average-size Tajik family, is equal to about $29 per person for the six-month course of treatment.

An evaluation of the scheme, from initiation in 2002 through the second quarter of 2004, compared treatment results of new patients registered in the program ($N = 459$) with a cohort that did not receive food support ($N = 39$). Results show the following:

—Cure rates were higher for the vulnerable group that received food support: 89.5 percent versus 59.4 percent,

—Treatment failure was 3.9 percent in the food support group versus 15.6 percent in the comparison cohort,

—2.9 percent of patients in the food support group died versus 12.5 percent in the comparison group,

—Default rates were considerably lower for the food support cohort: 3.7 percent versus 9.4 percent, and

—The program recognized that a larger-scale study is necessary to confirm positive findings.

Source: Mohr and others (2005); Mookherji and Beith (2005); Project HOPE/Tajikistan response to RPM Plus 2005 survey; personal correspondence, Tom Mohr, Tatyana Vinichenko, and Otabek Rajabov of Project HOPE/Tajikistan, June 2006.

part, increased case detection (90 percent compared with the national average of 82 percent) and cure rates (from 33 to 60 percent). This study did not distinguish the impact of the incentive, but it did find that the community-based approach to DOTS was more effective than the government's facility-based approach (Islam and others 2002; Mookherji and Beith 2005).

In India, the evaluation of a private provider payment scheme to refer suspected cases to microscopy centers and subsequently provide DOT revealed that case detection increased overall, the default rate was almost zero, and cure rates were the same as for public sector programs. These findings were attributed to a variety of factors that included the financial incentive.[8]

Evidence from DOTS and Providers

Evidence from routine monitoring data suggests that performance incentives for patients contribute to increased case detection and completion of treatment. In the Czech Republic, vouchers for material goods were given to homeless persons suspected of having tuberculosis who presented for testing. This resulted in case detection rates five times higher after the intervention.[9] It is possible, however, that because NGOs also receive an incentive for finding active cases, the increase in case detection might be in some part attributable to the patient incentive, the provider incentive, or both. In Romania, where support for patient travel was piloted, adherence increased to 95 percent. When the pilot program ended, rates decreased to 80 percent.[10] In Tajikistan, during periods when food support was not available, the patient default rate was 1.9 times higher than when food was available (Mohr and others 2005). In Moldova, food and hygienic articles may have been part of the reason for an increase in treatment success from 62 to 68 percent.[11]

On the provider side, findings from routine DOTS monitoring data also suggest that financial incentives contribute to improved performance. For example, in China, case-finding payments to village doctors may be behind increasing levels of case detection (Mookherji and Beith 2005). As mentioned, in the Czech Republic, NGOs received a case finding fee. This alone, or with the patient incentive, may have contributed to the fivefold increase in case detection rates.[12]

It is not possible to conclude unambiguously that performance incentives lead to better performance, although evidence from evaluations and from routine reporting do indicate promise. In addition, available evidence does not enable the impact of financial and material incentives to be separated from that of the

---

8. V. Inamdar in response to 2005 RPM Plus survey.

9. L. Trnka, National Tuberculosis Program, Czech Republic, in response to 2005 RPM Plus survey.

10. L. Ditiu, National Tuberculosis Program, Romania, in response to 2001 Stop TB, WHO, World Bank, and RPM Plus survey.

11. D. Laticevschi in response to 2005 RPM Plus survey.

12. L. Trnka, National Tuberculosis Program, Czech Republic, in response to 2005 RPM Plus survey.

package of other program-strengthening interventions that are implemented simultaneously.

Conclusions

Evidence of the contribution of performance incentives to increasing case detection and improving treatment completion rates suggests that incentives should be considered an integral element of a tuberculosis control strategy. For patients, financial or material incentives may be more effective when the transfer is conditional on some action correlated with tuberculosis control goals. For providers, performance incentives can be used in the public and private sector and at the individual and institutional levels. By understanding the existing environment within which the providers operate, we can design performance incentives to change behavior to achieve TB control goals.

Applying performance incentives to other disease interventions is also promising. Because treatment of drug-sensitive tuberculosis takes six to nine months, lessons about the impact of performance incentives to improve the results of TB programs may inform the management of other chronic health conditions. HIV/AIDS and TB are similar. They are communicable, effective treatment requires providing support to ensure patient adherence, and poor adherence can contribute to drug resistance. Noninfectious chronic conditions such as diabetes and hypertension also pose considerable challenges to patient adherence and the public health. Given commonalities in the service providers and mix of incentives, lessons about what motivates providers to diagnose and manage the treatment of tuberculosis can inform the design and implementation of these programs.

Experiences of performance-based incentive programs reveal key lessons for design and implementation:

—As part of the design process, consult with stakeholders to understand what motivates them.

—Consider how to communicate objectives of the program to the providers and patients who are both recipients and implementers.

—Include appropriate measures to track and monitor performance and put in place a process to assess and refine the approach as evidence is gathered and new lessons are learned.

—Anticipate potential complications of managing the distribution of money and food by studying challenges encountered in past programs.

Because the collection of routine monitoring data has been institutionalized in TB control programs around the world, program performance can be tracked on cases detected and treatment completed. This also facilitates comparison with national level information on performance and targets that have been established by the WHO. However, in both routine data and more rigorous studies, it is difficult to determine the unique contribution of performance incentives to improving the performance of tuberculosis programs because other interventions are implemented simultaneously. Although more evidence is needed on the precise impact of a menu of incentives, existing evidence suggests that carefully considered performance-based incentive programs can contribute to achieving TB program results.

References

Ambe, G., Knut Lönnroth, Y. Dholakia, J. Copreaux, M. Zignol, N. Borremans, and Mukund Uplekar. 2005. "Every Provider Counts: Effect of a Comprehensive Public-Private Mix Approach for TB Control in a Large Metropolitan Area in India." *International Journal of Tuberculosis and Lung Diseases* 9 (5): 562–68.

Beith, Alexandra, Rena Eichler, J. Sanderson, and Diana Weil. 2001. "Can Incentives and Enablers Improve the Performance of Tuberculosis Control Programs? Analytical Framework, Catalogue of Experiences, and Literature Review." Paper presented at the workshop Incentives and Enablers to Improve Performance of TB Control Programs, Paris, November 5–6.

Beith, Alexandra, P. Paredes, P. G. Suarez, and M. Thumm. 2004. "Workshop on the Use and Evaluation of Incentives in Tuberculosis Control in Latin America and the Caribbean: Trip Report, May 6–7, 2004." Report submitted to the U.S. Agency for International Development by the Rational Pharmaceutical Management Plus Program. Arlington, Va.: Management Sciences for Health.

Hanson, Christy L., Diana Weil, and Katherine Floyd. 2006. "Tuberculosis in the Poverty Alleviation Agenda." In *Reichman and Hershfield's Tuberculosis: A Comprehensive International Approach,* 3d ed., edited by Mario Raviglione. New York: Informa Healthcare USA.

Islam, M. Akramul, Susumu Wakai, Nobukatsu Ishikawa, A. M. R. Chowdhury, and J. Patrick Vaughan. 2002. "Cost-Effectiveness of Community Health Workers in Tuberculosis Control in Bangladesh." *Bulletin of the World Health Organization* 80 (6): 445–50.

Lönnroth, Knut. 2000. "Public Health in Private Hands." Ph.D. dissertation, University of Gothenburg.

Lönnroth, Knut, Mukund Uplekar, Vijay K. Arora, Sanjay Juvekar, Nguyen T. N. Lan, David Mwaniki, and Vikram Pathania. 2004. "Public-Private Mix for DOTS Implementation: What Makes It Work?" *Bulletin of the World Health Organization* 82 (8): 580–86.

Lönnroth, Knut, Mukund Uplekar, and Léopold Blanc. 2006. "Hard Gains through Soft Contracts: Productive Engagement of Private Providers in TB Control." *Bulletin of the World Health Organization* 84 (11): 876–83.

Midy, E., Y. Exume, and G. F. Celestin. 2004. "ICC-CAT: Projet de lutte contre la tuberculose avec assistance alimentaire et projet de recherches operationnelles; Evaluation finale." Unpublished manuscript. International Child Care.

Mohr, Tom, O. Rajobov, Z. Maksumova, and R. Northrup. 2005. "Using Incentives to Improve Tuberculosis Treatment Results: Lessons from Tajikistan." Millwood, Va.: CORE Tuberculosis Case Study and Project HOPE.

Mookherji, Sangeeta. 2005. "Impact and Cost-Effectiveness of Incentives and Enablers: Evidence and Policy Implications for TB Control Programmes?" Paper presented at the Thirty-Sixth World Congress. International Union Against Tuberculosis and Lung Disease, Paris, October.

Mookherji, Sangeeta, and Alexandra Beith. 2005. "Evaluating Tuberculosis Control Incentives and Enablers in the Context of Scale-up: Evidence and Experiences." Draft document for review. Arlington, Va.: Rational Pharmaceutical Management Plus Program, Management Sciences for Health.

Mookherji, Sangeeta, and Diana Weil. 2005. "Food Support to Tuberculosis Patients under DOTS: A Case Study of the Collaboration between the World Food Program and the National TB Control Program of Cambodia, December 8–17, 2002." Arlington, Va.: Management Sciences for Health and Stop TB Partnership.

Mookherji, Sangeeta, Diana Weil, Alexandra Beith, and C. Owunna. 2005. "Evaluating TB Enablers and Incentives Workshop Report: Paris, November 3–4, 2003." Report submitted to the U.S. Agency for International Development by the Rational Pharmaceutical Management Plus Program. Arlington, Va.: Management Sciences for Health and Stop TB Partnership.

Mookherji, Sangeeta, Diana Weil, M. T. Eang, and H. Mory. 2003. "Enabling TB Treatment Seeking and Completion through Food Support to Patients in Cambodia: A Case Study Approach." Paper presented at the Thirty-Fourth World Congress. International Union Against Tuberculosis and Lung Disease, Paris, October 29–November 2.

Nhlema, Bertha, and others. 2004. "A Systematic Analysis of TB and Poverty." Geneva: Stop TB Partnership, World Health Organization.

Stop TB/WHO (World Health Organization). 2006. "Actions for Life: Towards a World Free of Tuberculosis." Global Plan to Stop TB 1996–2015. Geneva: World Health Organization.

Town, Robert, and others. 2004. "Assessing the Influence of Incentives on Physicians and Medical Groups." *Medical Care Research and Review* 61 (3): S80–118.

Uplekar, Mukund W., S. D. Juvekar, D. B. Parande, D. B. Dalal, S. S. Khanvilkar, A. S. Vadair, and others. 1996. "Tuberculosis Management in Private Practice and Its Implications." *Indian Journal of Tuberculosis* 43 (1): 19–22.

Uplekar, Mukund, Vikram Pathania, and Mario Raviglione. 2001. "Involving Private Practitioners in Tuberculosis Control: Issues, Interventions, and Emerging Policy Framework." WHO document WHO/CDS/TB/2001.285. Geneva: World Health Organization.

WHO (World Health Organization). 2007. "WHO 2007 Tuberculosis Fact Sheet." Geneva. (www.who.int/mediacentre/factsheets/fs104/en/ [October 2008].)

Index

Acquired immunodeficiency syndrome (AIDS). *See* HIV/AIDS

ADB. *See* Asian Development Bank

Addiction. *See* Behavior and behavior modification

Administration. *See* Managers and management

Afghanistan: balanced scorecard, 150–52, 156, 158, 159; contracts and contracting in, 69, 141b, 142, 153–56, 157, 160, 161; European Commission and, 143–47, 149, 150t, 156, 158; FFSDP monitoring tool, 152–53, 161; Health Management Information System (HMIS) in, 149, 152, 154, 158, 159, 160, 162; history and health statistics of, 140–42, 153–56; loans to, 57; motivation of health workers in, 40, 161; monitoring and evaluating systems in, 149–60, 161; MoPH strengthening mechanism, 142, 150, 156, 156, 159; NGOs and donors in, 139–63; performance-based contracts and incen-

tives in, 41, 58, 62–63, 65, 87, 88, 139–40, 141, 142, 148, 149, 150t, 156–63; REACH program, 148, 149, 152, 153, 156, 161, 162, 163; stakeholder perceptions, 160–62; USAID and, 143–47, 148–49, 150t, 152, 158, 159, 161; World Bank and, 142–48, 149, 150, 156, 158, 160–61, 162, 163

Africa, 5, 12, 59, 238

African Development Bank, 193

Agreements. *See* Contracts and agreements

AIDS (acquired immunodeficiency syndrome). *See* HIV/AIDS

Americas, 12

Analyses, 53. *See also* Economic issues

Antoine, Uder, 165–88

Araujo, María Caridad, 93, 97

Argentina, 85, 90

Arrow, Kenneth, 17

Asia, 12, 238, 241

Asian Development Bank (ADB), 36, 141

Assessments and evaluations, 79–80, 81–85, 90–91, 134

Asthma, 34, 132
Ausila, Paul, 165–88

Bangladesh, 15, 28
Bangladesh Rural Advancement Committee,
	32, 243, 250, 252
Behavior and behavior modification: addic-
	tive behaviors, 33, 65, 126; in AIDS,
	malaria, and TB, 124, 128; chronic and
	noncommunicable conditions and, 14;
	conditionality and monitoring and,
	92–93, 97; different approaches to, 131;
	incentives and, 6, 7, 16, 18–20, 33, 59,
	125–30, 133–34; information and, 93;
	patient approaches to, 17; smoking, 19,
	33, 60, 123b, 124, 126–27, 128, 129,
	130; sustainability of behavior changes,
	33–34, 128, 132–33; in the United
	States, 123b, 134. See also Family plan-
	ning; Substance abuse
Beith, Alexandra, 237–56
Belgium Technical Cooperation (BTC),
	193, 194, 199–200, 204
Bolivia, 246
Bolsa Alimentação/Bolsa Familia (Brazil),
	90, 97, 99, 101t
Bono de Desarrollo Humano (Ecuador), 90
Botswana, 13
Boyce, Simone, 104, 108
Brazil, 30, 38, 39–40, 85, 101, 246
Bridges to Excellence, 29
BTC. See Belgium Technical Cooperation
Burden-of-disease analysis, 53
Butare, 210–13. See also Rwanda

Cambodia, 36, 68, 193, 243, 247, 248,
	249
Caribbean countries, 90
Case studies, 7b. See also Afghanistan; Haiti;
	Nicaragua; Rwanda; United States
Castro, Leslie, 108–09, 215–35
CCTs. See Conditional cash transfers
Centers for Disease Control (CDC), 130
Centres pour le Développement et la Santé
	(NGO), 167, 185
Chile, 85, 90

China, 14, 246, 253
Coady, David, 100
Colombia: CCT program in, 30, 32, 85,
	94, 96, 97, 101, 102, 103, 104t, 105t,
	106, 106, 107t, 109, 110, 111, 114;
	fertility in, 114; surveys in, 109–10
Comité Bienfaisance de Pignon (NGO),
	167, 185
Community-based organizations, 64
Competition. See Economic issues
Conditional cash transfers (CCTs): adminis-
	tration of, 67; age and, 106; assumptions
	of, 91–95, 105–06, 108, 116; conditions
	of, 92–93, 96–97, 98, 103, 106,
	114–15, 219; constraints of, 217; costs
	of, 101; demand- and supply-side fac-
	tors, 31–32, 35, 93–94, 102, 116, 117;
	design and goals of, 90, 91–102,
	114–15, 116–18; diet, calorie consump-
	tion, and nutrition, 106–08, 110–12;
	educational components of, 93–94, 96,
	106–07; eligibility and targeting, 97,
	99–100; evaluation and effects of, 27,
	31, 90, 94–95, 96, 102–18, 217; fertility
	and, 113–14; highlights of, 215b, 217;
	inefficiencies of, 92; monitoring and
	enforcement, 92–93, 96, 116; opera-
	tional arrangements, 101; payments/
	transfers of, 97, 99; program cycle, 96b;
	program effect model, 90–95; recipi-
	ents/beneficiaries of CCT resources, 60,
	93–94; spread of, 90; supply of services,
	108–09, 219; unintended effects of, 114,
	116; vaccination coverage under, 110.
	See also Performance incentives; Red de
	Protección Social; individual countries
Contingency management. See Managers
	and management
Contracts and agreements: assessment and
	evaluation of, 82–83; contract design, 18,
	67; donor and government restrictions,
	69–70; sample contract provisions,
	73–77, 81; unintended consequences
	and, 18, 19b
CORDAID, 193, 204
Costa Rica, 40, 90

Contributors

Uder Antoine
Management Sciences for Health

Paul Auxila
Management Sciences for Health

Alexandra Beith
Independent Consultant

Leslie Castro
Ministry of the Family, Nicaragua

Bernateau Desmangles
Management Sciences for Health

Rena Eichler
Broad Branch Associates

Gyuri Fritsche
Management Sciences for Health

Marie Gaarder
Inter-American Development Bank

Amanda Glassman
Inter-American Development Bank

Ruth Levine
Center for Global Development

Laurent Musando
World Health Organization

Natasha Palmer
*London School of Hygiene &
Tropical Medicine*

Mark Pauly
*Wharton School of the University of
Pennsylvania*

Ferdinando Regalia
Inter-American Development Bank

Louis Rusa
Ministry of Health, Rwanda

Miriam Schneidman
World Bank

Egbert Sondorp
*London School of Hygiene &
Tropical Medicine*

Lesley Strong
*London School of Hygiene &
Tropical Medicine*

Jessica Todd
American University

Kevin Volpp
*Wharton School of the University of
Pennsylvania*

Abdul Wali
*London School of Hygiene &
Tropical Medicine*

Diana Weil
World Health Organization